# READING
## AND
# WRITING
# CANCER

## ALSO BY SUSAN GUBAR

*Memoir of a Debulked Woman: Enduring Ovarian Cancer*

*True Confessions: Feminist Professors Tell Stories
Out of School*

*Judas: A Biography*

*Lo largo y lo corto del verso Holocausto*

*Feminist Literary Theory and Criticism*
(with Sandra M. Gilbert)

*Rooms of Our Own*

*Poetry After Auschwitz:
Remembering What One Never Knew*

*Critical Condition: Feminism at the Turn of the Century*

*Racechanges: White Skin, Black Face in American Culture*

*Masterpiece Theatre: An Academic Melodrama*
(with Sandra M. Gilbert)

*MotherSongs* (with Sandra M. Gilbert and Diana O'Hehir)

*English Inside and Out: The Places of Literary Criticism*
(with Jonathan Kamholtz)

*For Adults Users Only: The Dilemma of Violent Pornography*
(with Joan Hoff)

*No Man's Land, 3 vols.* (with Sandra M. Gilbert)

*The Norton Anthology of Literature by Women*
(with Sandra M. Gilbert)

*Shakespeare's Sisters: Feminist Essays on Women Poets*
(with Sandra M. Gilbert)

*The Madwoman in the Attic* (with Sandra M. Gilbert)

# READING
## AND
# WRITING
# CANCER

HOW WORDS HEAL

## Susan Gubar

W. W. NORTON & COMPANY

*INDEPENDENT PUBLISHERS SINCE 1923*

New York • London

For information about permission to reproduce selections from this book,
write to Permissions, W. W. Norton & Company, Inc.,
500 Fifth Avenue, New York, NY 10110

For information about special discounts for bulk purchases, please contact
W. W. Norton Special Sales at specialsales@wwnorton.com or 800-233-4830

Manufacturing by RR Donnelley Harrisonburg
Book design by Ellen Cipriano
Production manager: Louise Mattarelliano

ISBN 978-0-393-24698-8

W. W. Norton & Company, Inc.
500 Fifth Avenue, New York, N.Y. 10110
www.wwnorton.com

W. W. Norton & Company Ltd.
Castle House, 75/76 Wells Street, London W1T 3QT

1 2 3 4 5 6 7 8 9 0

For those who survive
and
those who do not

# Contents

PREFACE                                       1

CHAPTER 1
Coming to Terms                              11

CHAPTER 2
Impatient Memoirs                            58

CHAPTER 3
Sublime Artistry                            106

CHAPTER 4
My Blog                                     147

NOTES AND SUGGESTED READINGS                191

ACKNOWLEDGMENTS                             219

CREDITS                                     223

# READING
## AND
# WRITING
# CANCER

# Preface

D O WRITING AND READING about cancer right some of its grievous wrongs? In *Reading and Writing Cancer*, I answer this question with a resounding yes and then ask: why and how? I believe that engagement with cancer literature and art can alleviate the loneliness of the disease while enhancing our comprehension of how to grapple with it. These convictions arose from recent and not so recent personal experiences.

At the worst times, writing helps us remember. Only the paper napkins handed to me by a nurse enabled me to recall the moment I regained consciousness after the horrific debulking operation that ovarian cancer patients initially undergo. On the paper napkins I recorded my reactions to the rhythm of swabbing and swallowing: a morphine drip had chapped my lips and dried my mouth, and I spent the night with an oddly triangular plastic lollypop, a Styrofoam cup of ice chips . . . and the mounting pile of napkins. After that botched surgery in 2008 and throughout frightful reoperations and radiological procedures and cycles of chemotherapy, I always carried a pen and pad to record even the less dramatic protocols to which cancer patients are subjected. What would have been lost in a miasma of distress could be retrieved—with the preliminary and scanty jottings.

Although in my previous book, *Memoir of a Debulked Woman*, I recounted medical treatments that seemed worse than the disease, using my notes and writing the manuscript helped me immeasurably: not only to recall the gruesome events I had endured, but also to serve as a patient-advocate, protesting the so-called gold standard of treatment. More, the process of composition turned out to be as uplifting and inspiring for me as meditation is for others: a way of steadying myself, gaining perspective, quieting anxieties, and shifting my attention from my ailing body to words, to sentences, and (best of all) to the experiences of other people. For between drafting and revising, I avidly devoured accounts composed by men and women confronting different cancers. "In illness," Virginia Woolf believed, "words seem to possess a mystic quality."

For the past two years, I have been kept alive by a clinical trial and by the *New York Times*. The regular appearance of my blog, "Living with Cancer," has been as life-enhancing for me as the packets of an experimental drug I receive at the Indiana University Simon Cancer Center. Actually, because I have control over the drafting and revising of the essays, they play an even more miraculous role than the pills in revitalizing my existence. This venture has convinced me that writing is an effective complementary therapy for cancer patients coping with the consequences of a ghastly disease.

At the same time, doing research for the blogs has persuaded me that reading the vibrant works of others eases the anxiety of cancer and clarifies what we are going through individually. Now that I have been granted the benefits of a less debilitating targeted drug in a clinical trial, I am able to reflect on these processes. In my absorption with words, I resemble many patient-writers, who have produced journals, poems, graphic memoirs, op-ed columns, sociological books, and performance pieces to challenge and change medical protocols; to help heal, fortify, or renew themselves; and to forge an ongoing cancer canon.

*Reading and Writing Cancer* explores a unique phenomenon in contemporary times: an explosion of responses to a particular group of diseases not by medical specialists (who have been writing about cancer for centuries) but by patients, caregivers, and artists. For the most part, their work is personally expressive rather than scientific, historical, policy-driven, or polemical. Diaries, essays, memoirs, short stories, and novels—as well as photographs, paintings, movies, television series, and blogs—play a major role today in shaping public understanding of various cancers. Taken together, these productions establish an evolving tradition that has not yet been recognized or charted. I begin by describing writing as a form of therapy and then consider how patients and caregivers, as well as people I am tempted to call civilians or bystanders, have made use of a range of inventive forms that can stimulate and solace us during hard times.

Obviously, writing cannot cure patients, but it facilitates the progress of repairing the damages done. Words have the power to mend spirits abiding within damaged or incurable bodies. Yet some authors of cancer narratives, in thinking about their productions, would undoubtedly object to the term "therapy," since it can feel frightening and painful, rather than restorative, to examine the catastrophic repercussions of a cancer diagnosis and its resultant treatments. Like many responding to trauma, such writers would instead describe what they were doing as testifying or bearing witness. Others, especially self-defined artists, might feel that the word "therapy" erases the rigorous craft involved in framing evocative structures, metaphors, scenes, and arguments to heighten the effect of their productions.

However, therapy is commonly defined as rigorous as well as painful work. Even when engaged in the labor of crafting, or of testifying and bearing witness, cancer patients frequently find that writing about the disease eventually performs a therapeutic function, especially if they have experienced themselves as robbed of who they were before diagnosis or, worse yet, evacuated of any sense of self during treatment.

Surgery, radiation, and chemotherapy can cause patients to feel so invaded, so bombarded, so infused that they lose a sense of their own agency, of subjectivity, even of language. The writing process enables a reconstitution of the self—probably not the same self that existed before diagnosis, but nevertheless another authentic self and a voice. Be it angry or sorrowful, defiant or resigned, courageous or fearful, this emergent voice helps us understand who we are becoming.

With its eccentric intonation, diction, and rhythm, what we call the voice in the silence of writing can quite distinctively identify a unique individual. (Its potential for singularity reminds me of friends who need only say on the phone "Hi, do you have a minute?" and I know exactly who is calling.) The writing process, in its creation of an exterior expression of the self, resembles other therapeutic activities available to people whose physical strength is impaired: painting, for example, or playing an instrument. But of course most of us learn the basics of composition in our early education, while fewer acquire the rudiments of the visual and musical arts—which is why writing has attained such a prominent role in patients' reactions to cancer.

This book addresses people who want to write more effectively about the impact of disease on their lives as well as people who want to read or view works that—through their crafty artifice—instruct us on the physical, mental, emotional, social, and economic repercussions of various cancers and treatments. By reading some-times disturbing writing or viewing sometimes perplexing artwork about cancer, we can discover multiple ways to live with the disease. The first and last chapters of this book discuss writing, the middle two reading. Of course, brilliant representations of breast cancer abound; however, I have made every effort to include as well work that addresses cancer arising from a number of other organs and pathways.

Although I do not reprint any of my *New York Times* essays in their entirety, I amplify my responses to a number of the issues I encountered while doing my research for them. Sometimes material in this book migrated into the blog and sometimes passages in the blog migrated into this book. In the last chapter, an autobiograph-ical essay, I reflect on the problems and pleasures of blogging and incorporate some drafted posts that I never dared to submit. Before that conclusion, the chapters of this book progress from the least to the most complex forms of composition, but all were designed to stand alone and can be read out of order. Indeed, each is composed from a different perspective, for I start out as a writing coach and then I draw on my experience as a memoirist, a literary critic, and finally a blogger.

In the first chapter, "Coming to Terms," I discuss the bene-fits of so-called free writing and diaries. Here I summarize medical research showing that expressive composition improves the lives of cancer patients psychologically and also physiologically. Since the rudiments of journal writing have been established and taught for decades, I apply them to the context of cancer by providing a series of writing prompts, describing a number of well-established rou-tines and exercises, and proposing models for imitation.

The second chapter, "Impatient Memoirs," asks: What do we gain from reading accounts of profoundly private experiences that have been transformed into public testimonials of the body under siege? Within the conventional structure of the cancer memoir, patients and caregivers criticize medical practices, imagine the nature of cancer, and confront the injuries brought about by both. In innovative reinventions of the memoir form, humorists and graphic artists, as well as ecological and spiritual thinkers, have produced absorbing depictions of the fraught and yet fertile psychic geography navigated by patients.

The adjective in the title of chapter 3, "Sublime Artistry," refers to disturbing but fascinating art composed about (but not necessarily by) people dealing with cancer. Creative artists who attend to the suffering caused by cancer produce awe-inspiring photographs, stories, paintings, plays, and novels, especially when they postulate the unexpected possibility of deathbed sublimity. Artistic representations of cancer—unsettling for readers or viewers—repel us with their visceral portrayal of an implacable threat to our existence, and yet they also attract us with a sense that by contemplating such a threat we at least partly confront and possibly comprehend or accept it.

Moving from the sublime to the quotidian in chapter 4, *Reading and Writing Cancer* concludes with a personal essay about my blog. Cancer patients have gained enormously from the Web's up-to-the-minute reports and from its potential to put people into communication networks, but does the medium of the blog pose unique challenges? Here I address the issue of audience by touching on the complicated ethics of self-revelation. How is it possible to write truthfully about intimate experiences without embarrassing ourselves or marginalizing others? For people like me who do decide to risk at least some self-exposure, I suggest a number of formats to generate and enrich the composition of short essays.

Taken together, the chapters of this book demonstrate that we are observing and participating in a fundamental change in the world of letters. In the 1920s, Virginia Woolf decried the paucity of literature about sickness: "illness has not taken its place with love and battle and jealousy among the prime themes of literature." According to Woolf, authors up to her day preferred to concern themselves with the mind, whereas in illness the body predominates. However, the contemporary works I have found suggest that disease is starting to take its place among the prime themes of literature. The most intriguing of them put into play two fundamentally antagonistic categories: writing, which seeks to enlighten or entertain, and cancer, which is just about the least enlightening or entertaining topic that most people can conceive of. In the process of meditating on the relationship of writing to cancer, the authors of these texts tell us about the power as well as the impotence of literature, even as they stir us with their discernment.

Throughout I have sought to create a mix between a manual and a map: a manual for those who want to write, a map for those who want to read and view. Actually, I wanted to produce a sketchy manual and map, rather than an elaborately detailed or definitive one. Whenever I imagined this volume, it was slim because cancer patients and their caregivers have to meet so many obligations—urgent physical crises, regular medical appointments, family quandaries, money problems—that they do not have time to slog through an expansive disquisition. Nor did I know how long I would be physically well enough to concentrate on the composition.

I am also aware that we reside in the midst of the development of the cancer canon. Although occasionally I look back on early historical periods, most of the works discussed in this book were created after the 1970s, when cancer ceased to be a monolithic term and began to be treated as a group of differentiated and quite distinct diseases. During the turn into the twenty-first century, the paternalism of the medical establishment diminished as more women entered the profession. Patient empowerment movements sprang up as medical information became democratized, and doctors began to disclose prognoses and treatment consequences more truthfully. All of these changes—affecting the cancer canon and effected by it—occurred while the demarcation between public discourse and private lives continued to erode. In our time, we can only surmise what contours this tradition will take.

*Reading and Writing Cancer* is therefore not an encyclopedic overview of everything that has been thought and said about cancer writing. Indeed, some genres—children's literature, poetry—receive little attention. For the most part, I deal with texts decidedly focused on cancer, although the disease has impelled writers to produce all sorts of works on every conceivable subject. Many of the jaunty self-help books and articles that are commercially successful—works imbued with the power of positive thinking or enforcing what one critic calls "the tyranny of cheerfulness"—I have left for the sociologists who study ongoing evidence of Americans' optimistic faith in the power of their individualism.

Even for those forms that I found particularly important, I have often chosen a representative text to stand for a host of others, rather than surveying everything that has been published. For visual works, I point readers toward Web locations so that they can see the paintings, photographs, and cartoons on the screen. I'm quite certain I have missed important works and will kick myself at having left them out, but none of us are specialists yet on this subject and I will learn from all the omissions that readers discover.

Since each chapter addresses a subject that could be a book on its own, I have had to condense quite a bit. At the back of the volume, notes to chapters supply the page citations for passages I have quoted and include further suggested readings and occasionally scholarly background material. These endnotes are keyed to pages rather than note numbers to reduce the risk of distracting the reader. To provide a diversion from tendentious advice books, I have attempted to present not an argument about the proper way to deal with cancer but rather a guide to a broad spectrum of responses displaying how people from various perspectives and with diverse values and experiences have reacted to a succession of treatments or the disease's progress.

The roads surveyed on this map often take hazardous turns. But by setting out together, we can learn to negotiate the terrain, glimpse less painful and more productive routes, relish companionship along the way, and help teach the experts—physicians and nurses, social workers and health care advocates—what patients need on our various journeys. In these pages, cancer patients can get to know fellow travelers who have abundant insights to share.

I have been teaching and writing about writing for some fifty years and will draw on that background throughout the coming pages. But this project has entranced me like no other—perhaps because it comes from the core of my being, the center of my heart. Whereas cancer has been the bane of my life, writing has been its boon. Although cancer remains a depressing subject, writing aims at enlightenment and, when possible, delight. As did many of the writers discussed in the pages to come, I have decided that if we have to have cancer, we can put it to use. I rejoice in the prospect that readers will put this book to good use.

When my essays started to appear in the online *New York Times,* I thought it was ironic that they were coming out in a section called "Well." Increasingly, though, I have realized that even while dealing with an incurable condition, I can find springs and founts of pleasure. Composing this book has furnished quite a few of those. I hope it and the practices of writing and reading and looking that it describes will become a source of healing: a deep and somewhat scary but nonetheless refreshing well in the world.

# Chapter 1

# Coming to Terms

IT IS A TRUTH generally acknowledged that a person dispossessed of health must be in want of paper and pen or a computer—and lots of books. All sorts of fictional and nonfictional works deliver solace and pleasure to the ailing, but books about cancer inspire writing about cancer, which in turn enables patients to understand what we are experiencing. "How can I tell what I think till I see what I say?" the novelist E. M. Forster once asked. How can I tell what I think about disease until I see what I write?

The art of great writing cannot be taught, but the craft of expressive writing can certainly be learned. Over the past few decades, a number of well-established activities and exercises—developed by composition teachers—have been used to transform beginners into devoted and supple authors of difficult passages in their life stories. They can easily be adapted to and adopted by people dealing with cancer. The loneliness, boredom, exasperation, anxiety, and enervation of treatments can be greatly alleviated by the act of writing and by reading that prompts more writing.

Should you be in the large population of people grappling with some sort of cancer, perhaps you were lucky and your disease was caught at an early stage, but perhaps not. Whether you have lost a breast or a testicle, a chunk of lung or liver, or simply but shockingly your assurance in your future well-being, you have had to deal with the abrupt threat of your impending mortality. For many of us, distress at confronting the vulnerability and transience of existence may have been exacerbated by the physical and psychological injuries associated with surgery, radiation, and chemotherapy. In quite a few patients, cancer and its treatments spawn depression over grievous losses. This chapter—composed for people with any type or stage of cancer and for those who seek to support them—proposes and explores writing as an alternative therapy that can benefit all of us enduring the bruising jolt of a cancer diagnosis and the damages that treatment may bring in its wake.

After a diagnosis of late-stage ovarian cancer in 2008, I underwent three abdominal surgeries, three cycles of chemotherapies, and umpteen radiological procedures, conventional medical regimens that made me miserable. Yet I remained and remain allergic to most alternative approaches to disease . . . on quirky, not rational, grounds.

I am afraid of needles—too many have been stuck into me in hospitals—so I have never tried acupuncture. I am fearful of strangers touching me—another problem in hospitals—so I never signed up for massage or healing hands. I fidget and worry and wander when trying to sit still and meditate. Visualization unfortunately brings apocalyptic images to mind. I distrust potions and lotions unregulated by the FDA, and therefore mistletoe injections and cappuccino enemas do not appear on my to-do lists. When not nauseated or weakened by treatment, I revel in an appetite for any sort of food (and the strength to cook it), so I refrain from macrobiotic or vegan or other restrictive diets. Given this obstinate stance, how can I propose writing as an alternative therapy?

From 2008 until I enlisted in a Phase I clinical trial in 2012, I was too weak to engage in physical exercise, but I could sit lengthwise on the blue couch in my living room with my legs outstretched and a laptop perched on them. My body was resting, as it needed to do, but my fingers did the walking: taking me to many websites where other patients asked and answered questions about cancer, engaging me in lively email conversations with family and friends, and affording me the opportunity to record my feelings and thoughts about the diminishment of my life.

During perilous times—after a surgery or in the foggy fatigue following chemotherapy—I might only list my medications or the dates of upcoming appointments. After the staples were removed or when the fog momentarily lifted, though, I could describe the arctic, antic zones of the hospital. Often, then, mundane descriptions would pique my attention, somehow snagging my interest, and I would start to elaborate on the zany hats and New Age music in the freezing operating room or the periodic chimes announcing new births as I reclined cocooned within a warmed blanket in the chilly infusion unit.

Because writing is sedentary, because it can be done anywhere, intermittently, by anyone, because it is cheap and need not involve a computer but can easily be accomplished with a pad and pencil, because it requires no other people, and because writing breeds writing, it remains one of the few productive activities available to many cancer patients. People facing cancer often must relinquish domestic and professional responsibilities and therefore have time in which we can consider and convert our losses into the gains of understanding maybe not the disease itself but our own evolving condition. There are, of course, the blocks that all writers confront, as well as specific obstacles that patients encounter. However, when they can be circumvented, writing becomes a restorative activity that supplements standard medical responses to cancer.

In some respects, the writing process resembles the only other complementary intervention I have found beneficial. I joined a yoga class for cancer patients after conventional medical care concluded and I started receiving a targeted drug in a clinical trial. Daily pills (taken at home) do not wreak the havoc of chemotherapy (infused in the hospital), so I have the energy needed for the cats-and-cows, the tree and warrior poses, and (my personal favorite) the supine pigeon, undertaken at the local YMCA. Although gentle yoga requires more anatomical flexibility than does writing, it instills some of the same benefits: relaxation, steadiness, a stilling of nattering voices in the brain, a sense of balance, strength, and achievement.

The stretches and postures of yoga emphasize the body, while the stretches and postures of writing exercise the mind. But like meditation, yoga and writing can be undertaken in silent solitude; and both can suspend time, instilling respect for oneself, for others, and for the universe. What they promote is mindfulness, a word tarnished by too much self-help hype but one that nevertheless gestures toward a quiet state of attentiveness.

Truth be told, sometimes when I am in the grip of a writing venture, the adrenaline coursing through me makes me feel way more hyped than yogic. My insistent need to write is hardly anomalous. "The fact of having cancer," the psycho-oncologist Esther Dreifuss-Kattan attests, "can evoke in many patients a strong wish for self-expression."

To address this powerful desire for self-expression, I set out here first to define writing therapy and to briefly summarize research proving it to be beneficial for patients. Then I suggest some specific techniques that coaches have used for decades to facilitate so-called free writing and what is unfortunately called "journaling," a verb I promise to abjure from now on. Next this chapter turns to exemplary diarists of the past whose strategies provide models for both beginning and seasoned writers. Finally, I sketch some standard principles of revision. But throughout I try to keep in mind that the writing process may change for people in treatment. When we lose words in the fog of chemotherapy, when we lose concentration because of the rashes or burns of radiation, when we lose strength from surgical wounds, when we lose the use of hands and feet frozen or numbed from neuropathy, when we lose appetite and libido, it may be difficult for us to imagine sustaining any activity at all.

In her brilliant poem "One Art," Elizabeth Bishop declares over and over again that the art of losing is not too hard to master, though she sounds like she herself needs convincing. For it *is* hard to master loss; at times, it may be impossible. Yet she tells herself that practice makes perfect, that she need only start with small losses, like a lost hour or her mother's watch, before she will be able to withstand bigger losses, like the loss of her home or her homeland. At the close of the poem, when Bishop thinks about losing the most beloved person in her life, she stammers at the prospect of inconsolable bereavement: "the art of losing's not too hard to master / though it may look like (*Write* it!) like disaster."

The repetition of the word "like" before and after the parenthetical command informs us of Bishop's stuttering, gasping pain, but also of the urgency of finding an analogy through which she can understand her suffering. Even and perhaps especially during times of loss, we may need to urge ourselves to "*Write* it." For writing provides a way not necessarily to master disaster, but to comprehend and accept or contend with it.

Writing therapy often starts out spontaneously, as it did for me when I first met my oncologist, Dr. Matei. To prepare for that meeting, I assembled a list of questions about the prognosis of my disease and the chemotherapy regimen. The social skills of the surgeon earlier assigned to me had left something to be desired. A number of my inquiries were therefore aimed at discovering whether Dr. Matei and I could communicate freely with each other. Throughout our conversation, I tried to jot down notes so I could remember exactly what she said about the pathology report, the drugs she would pre-scribe, their potential side effects, and the number of sessions in the first cycle of infusions. She turned out to be not only a charming person but also a truth-teller, much to my delight.

Unlike some patients who quite understandably resist knowing their statistical odds and unlike others who quite understandably could not care less about the personality of their doctor, I wanted the hard facts and relished their being delivered by a captivating young woman whose mordant sense of humor had been molded by the Romanian culture she had fled. That she was a poet sealed the deal.

Even such a mundane example, a list of questions, exemplifies the nature and benefits of the writing process. A list or notes jot-ted down before a medical consultation focuses the mind, expresses concerns or anxieties, and conveys priorities as well as values. For me, and for others, it may be impossible to know what is in my mind, what concerns and anxieties hold sway, which priorities and values I am bringing into an important conversation unless I write them down. For some of us, as E. M. Forster believed, writing really is a way of thinking and feeling and learning about ourselves: a mode of introspection. Without it, we are at sea.

"Language is the mother of thought, not the handmaiden of thought," the poet W. H. Auden once said, quoting an Austrian aphorist, and then he added, "words will tell you things you never thought or felt before." The novelist Judith Guest put it this way: "writers do not write to *impart* knowledge to others; rather, they write to *inform* themselves." Joan Didion composes autobiographical essays "entirely to find out what I'm thinking, what I'm looking at, what I see and what it means."

If this is the case for many under ordinary circumstances, consider the impact of a cancer diagnosis. It can arrive like a thudding blow, a lightning bolt, an exploding bomb, a crack opening up in the earth beneath our feet. Or it can arrive like an icy chill, the blank numbness of disbelief, since not-knowing may seem preferable to believing and comprehending that one's life will never be the same as it was before. Or, oddly, it can arrive, as it did for me, with relief at finally understanding what is wrong, followed by crippling trepidation about what to do about it. Hearing a diagnosis is, in other words, a shock, an injury . . . and a threshold: one stage of life has closed; another is opening. We wander between two worlds, one extinct and the other frightfully unpredictable.

For this reason, some people—years, even decades after diagnosis—keep in mind their "cancerversaries": the annual recurrence of the date of their discovery of the type and stage of their cancer. Because cancer undoubtedly existed in the body before its detection, the diagnosis date always feels belated and faintly fictive; however, it marks a disruptive discontinuity in consciousness. Like a wedding or death anniversary, the cancerversary commemorates an end and a beginning—in this case a traumatic beginning.

After dealing with testicular cancer, the sociologist Arthur W. Frank "wanted less to recover what I had been than to discover what else I might be. Writing is part of this discovery." Composition may play several roles not only after but also during treatment for patients as well as caretakers who want to understand their post-diagnosis world. A chorus of voices substantiates this point.

While getting hormonal injections for metastatic prostate cancer, Anatole Broyard explained, "Writing is a counterpoint to my illness. It forces the cancer to go through my character before it can get to me." Toward the end of seven weeks of radiation and chemotherapy for adenoid cystic carcinoma that had spread from his tongue to his neck and lungs, Matt Freedman could not speak and could swallow only liquids; but filling a sketchbook with his diary entries and drawings—four pages a day—became a sustaining routine as practical as symptom monitoring and calorie counting: "the book is helping me get through this."

During an autologous bone marrow transplant for relapsed Hodgkin's disease, Dan Shapiro discovered that "writing of my experiences brushes a healing balm of perspective on them. I understand what I want and what I don't want." John Diamond considered his memoir "part of my cure" of throat and oral cancers: "Or if not that, then part of my reconciliation with the fact that whatever happens I will live with cancer for the rest of my life, and with the understanding that this doesn't mean there aren't still a few good times to come." Le Anne Schreiber kept a day-by-day record of her mother's last months with pancreatic cancer; it became "my means of survival," a reminder that "I was a witness to dying, not the one dying," and a "weapon against denial."

To my mind, any and all sorts of writing that engages patients and caregivers contending with cancer—whether or not its content centers on the disease—constitutes writing therapy, though others define it more narrowly. Psychologists have argued for quite some time that expressive writing can help heal people dealing with the shock of death, domestic violence, and historical as well as natural calamities. During the last decades of the twentieth century, the pioneering psychologist James W. Pennebaker undertook experiments with students, building on growing evidence that "translating events into language can affect brain and immune function."

Pennebaker divided one early group of volunteers in two, with the first group writing about traumatic experiences and the second about superficial topics. Then the first group was divided into three: those who described their emotions during the writing sessions, those who wrote only about the facts of trauma, and those who wrote about the facts and their emotional reactions to their traumas. This last group profited most, according to Pennebaker: "People who wrote about their deepest thoughts and feelings surrounding a trauma evidenced an impressive drop in illness visits after the study compared with the other groups."

In *Opening Up: The Healing Power of Expressing Emotions*, Pennebaker summarized the findings of dozens of writing experiments: "Writing about emotional upheavals has been found to improve the physical and mental health of grade-school children, maximum security prisoners, new mothers, and rape victims." Louise DeSalvo based her guide *Writing as a Way of Healing* on Pennebaker's findings. She imagines writing as a sort of fixer, like the chemicals used to stabilize a photographic image. A writing instructor who decades ago taught a class at Hunter College that, fortuitously, my mother audited, DeSalvo invites her students "to use writing as a way of healing, as a fixer, as a sturdy ladder, as picking and digging, as balm on a wound—or whatever metaphor describes how the process works for you." With the help of various writing programs, veterans of recent wars and people with a range of mental illnesses have produced memoirs that reflect on the lifeline furnished by the process of composition.

For my mother, whose family had been devastated by Hitler's rise to power, the chronicle she began in Louise DeSalvo's classroom enabled her to mourn her dead parents, in-laws, aunts, uncles, and cousins, while memorializing them for her grandchildren and their children. As numerous scholars in trauma studies have shown, Anne Frank, Elie Wiesel, and Primo Levi used witnessing as a political act to protest injury and also as a psychological process that helped them deal with grievous circumstances. In a genocidal context, exorcism or catharsis may be impossible for many, and yet, one hopes, not for all.

When Jeffrey Wolin produced a series of photographs of Holocaust survivors, he inscribed their first-person testimonies on the black-and-white portraits because he believed these accounts served as a bridge, conveying survivors from a disastrous European past into a secure American present. Of course "Cancer is not a concentration camp," the doctor-author Siddhartha Mukherjee knows, "but it shares the quality of annihilation: it negates the possibility of life outside and beyond itself; it subsumes all living. The daily life of a patient becomes so intensely preoccupied with his or her illness that the world fades away."

Esther Dreifuss-Kattan's psychoanalytic approach in *Cancer Stories: Creativity and Self-Repair* makes the case for writing as beneficial specifically to cancer patients. This book traces creativity back to the sort of play that involves children with transitional objects (a blanket, a teddy bear); such play enables babies to grapple with fears of maternal abandonment: "As the transitional object in infancy could be used as a symbol for the absent mother, the cancer book, poem, or picture can become the mediating symbol of separation and togetherness, of dying and immortality." Like painting or sculpting, writing functions as a creative defense against present and future losses. According to Dreifuss-Kattan, "writing the cancer book or painting the cancer picture is a powerful alternative to more primitive responses" such as denial or rage or depression. A literary or artistic endeavor helps people with cancer confront separation, mourn their losses, and "establish a relationship to the new realities they are forced to face."

The specifics of one scientific study can exemplify empirical research on writing as cancer therapy. In the March 1, 2014, issue of the *Journal of Clinical Oncology*, Dr. Kathrin Milbury and other researchers published an article on a randomized writing trial. Four 20-minute sessions of expressive writing improved outcomes for patients with all stages of renal cell carcinoma. Some 200 patients at MD Anderson were divided into two groups, with half doing "neutral writing" (about everyday topics) and half plumbing their feelings about difficult experiences related to cancer.

Follow-up tests proved that those who engaged in writing about their emotions suffered less depression and fatigue, and fewer sleep disorders and quality of life problems. Researchers found that "the most pronounced group differences emerged 10 months after the intervention." Building on previous studies on writing therapy that enrolled women with breast cancer, the investigators conclude, "We demonstrated that EW [expressive writing] seems to be equally beneficial for men and women with RCC [renal cell carcinoma]."

EW hardly looks or sounds like a tempting acronym. But expressive writing that involves people wrestling with their profound responses to disease does need to be contrasted with dutifully plunking down words on such topics as the weather last week. In other words, penciling and then penciling again the sentence "All work and no play makes Jack a dull boy" is not going to help even the likes of Jack Nicholson. (Isn't *The Shining* the greatest horror movie about writing ever?)

Because researchers have shown that expressive writing or journal therapy boosts the physical and mental health of cancer patients, writing programs abound at many hospitals where trained mentors—teachers, editors, journalists—offer prompts, cues, and feedback, often at no or minimal cost. Visible Ink, a free program at Memorial Sloan-Kettering, pairs patients with experienced mentors; publishes an annual anthology of poems, plays, and essays; and uses seasoned actors, dancers, and singers to stage an annual performance of composed works. Anne Hunsaker Hawkins, who supervises medical students involved with patient writing projects at the Penn State College of Medicine, believes that "the possibility of an audience of readers" makes the act of composition meaningful. For people like me, without the energy to travel or interact with strangers, only a pad and pencil (or their electronic equivalent) are needed, perhaps together with some of the practices proposed in the rest of this chapter.

A number of skeptical specialists have warned that writing may be therapeutic, but it is not therapy. If they mean that writing must not be confused with or undertaken instead of psychoanalysis or other forms of talk therapy, they surely have a point. However, since the time of Sigmund Freud, psychoanalysts have associated a fractured life narrative with mental illness, the emergence of a coherent life narrative with mental health. And in the past few years, psychologists have proven that people who are encouraged to redirect the stories they tell about themselves can improve their self-perceptions. Other specialists, more critical, caution that writers can become neurotically self-regarding, thereby perpetuating the injuries suffered. Yet even professional authors, notorious for their overweening narcissism, have found writing salutary in coping with life's little ironies.

Addressing an audience of surgeons, the commercially successful author Rudyard Kipling said, "Words are, of course, the most powerful drug used by mankind." The novelist Graham Greene believed that "writing is a form of therapy; sometimes I wonder how all those who do not write, compose or paint can manage to escape the madness, the melancholia, the panic fear which is inherent in the human situation."

The easiest way to start and sustain writing for many people happens through a process Peter Elbow made famous—so-called free writing—and involves keeping a diary. Instead of assuming that you need to figure out what you want to say and outlining your ideas before beginning, would-be writers are more successful when they start writing immediately—without knowing what they are setting out to communicate. Meaning emerges through the process itself. Some instructors call this automatic writing and claim that it lets people "bypass the head and ego and write straight from the heart." Others believe that it liberates adults from early miseducation that inculcated inhibiting and punitive self-judgments. "Not being able to write," according to the writing teacher Pat Schneider, "is almost always the result of scar tissue, of disbelief in yourself accumulated as a result of unhelpful responses to your writing."

Proponents of free writing encourage people to allocate a specific part of the day and spend a specific amount of time, say 20 minutes, taking risks by recording whatever comes to mind without checking grammar or spelling, without stopping to correct or revise. After you have purchased a notebook or set up a computer file for your diary, the point is to keep on filling up the page or screen with sentences, even if they seem jagged or junky or jerky, and not to get up and clean the refrigerator or walk the dog. "Writing badly is a crucial part of learning to write well," Elbow reminds us.

Sometimes people who sit down to record the events of the day or reflect upon them feel in need of a nudge. Instructors of free writing provide students with prompts that can easily be translated into cues for cancer patients. One type of prompt serves as an assignment for a single day's session. Here are some I have devised.

Describe the radiology mask or the catheter attached to your body.

Untie the strands of a domestic or work-related knot created by treatment.

Remember the moment of diagnosis or of telling a sibling about it.

Visualize what your cancer or your fear looks like.

Brood over a worst-case or best-case scenario of an upcoming biopsy or scan.

Weigh the consequences of two alternative proposed medical protocols.

Draft a letter to someone you want in or out of your life.

Itemize the equipment, pills, paraphernalia you have acquired.

Imagine a family occasion without you.

Pretend you are your partner or your child dealing with your condition.

Record a conversation at your cancer support group meeting.

Interview a health care professional.

Celebrate or castigate a doctor or nurse.

Summarize or respond to a cancer essay.

Listen to a piece of music you love and write down your
responses.

Contemplate your attitudes toward genetic testing.

Consider your dietary or exercise goals.

Invent a landscape or a metaphor for nausea, fatigue, pain,
or a drug's effect.

Create a prayer or a curse.

Another type of prompt to initiate writing functions as the start of a sentence. A springboard, it gives you a beginning that you can complete. Here are some I've come up with, though you can easily devise your own.

I wish I could tell my oncologist . . .

My friend responded to my cancer by . . .

Today, or yesterday, I found myself puzzled or inspired
by . . .

In my experience, the financial cost of cancer . . .

The side effect I would never have expected surfaced as . . .

After researching the clinical trial, I think . . .

As a caregiver with cancer, I understand that . . .

Waking at 3 a.m., I . . .

I used to . . . , but now I . . .

When I sit in the waiting room . . .

My spiritual practice has begun to include . . .

I am not yet ready to confront . . .

Before next year, I want to . . .

My energy during treatment has been . . .

When I look in the mirror, I see . . .

What takes my mind off disease is . . .

Ironically, cancer has brought into my life . . .

In my most snarky mood, I attribute the cause of my disease
to . . .

From my perspective, healthy people seem very . . .


The greatest benefit of automatic writing is its freedom of expression, since it is meant for your eyes only. Here is a place to articulate fears or hopes that might be inexpressible to others, to linger over a truth that you have discovered about your situation or your feelings about it. If you take on one of these assignments and get stuck, pretend that a friend has inquired about the topic or related his experiences, asking you to share yours.

You might want to devote two or more different sessions of free writing to one single prompt in order to see what you have to say. Peter Elbow calls this "cooking" and "growing" your prose, which you can then reread to grasp its central point and to edit: to sum it up with a simple assertion, cut out dead wood, and find the better word. Through this process—a few days or even weeks or months later—your sentences may become a draft for a shapely letter or personal essay. Or your prose—whether or not revised for concision, coherence, grammar, and style—can retain its immediacy and be left as is in a private journal.

For another group of people, especially those who have done quite a bit of writing in the past, sometimes writing that is less free— should we call it compulsive writing?—might come more naturally, as it does for me. I know I am a compulsive writer because I cannot stop myself from rewriting while I am in the midst of writing. A sentence or two arrives in a spurt, and then rereading and revising lead to another. Often in my diary, very often, I simply recount my day. Sometimes, though, I have an urgent concern when I open my diary computer file, scroll to the end, and fill in the date.

If I have a clear sense of a current problem I want to address, I make an outline—(1) an instance of forgetfulness, (2) words I have misread, (3) thoughts I have forgotten, (4) social embarrassments— through which I gain a sense of the purpose of the writing, which may be a few pages long. Since I am a compulsive, not a free, writer, even at this preliminary stage I take to heart the credo shared by Mark Twain and many surgeons: when in doubt, cut it out. If a title pops into mind—"Chemo Bane"—I mull over what I might make of it in another writing session, for a provisional title focuses me and a journal entry may eventually morph into an essay.

Even and perhaps especially compulsive writers confront with horror the nauseating bilge that spills out onto the screen or the page. I look at my two pathetic sentences about instances of chemo brain and think: so what, who cares? Or I think: they can't possibly capture my sense of befuddlement. But then their very failure to really encapsulate what genuinely upsets me about my current condition leads me to multiply examples, and then those, in turn, absorb my attention. If I don't make the effort now, I realize, the experience will be lost.

And given my chemo brain, I will never remember when the youngest grandbaby first smiled—it was captured in an October 24, 2014, photo—if I don't write it down. So I force myself to note my mixed response to dear friends leaving town for a better job or my worries about my husband's backache or a daughter's battle with head lice; I will be able to reread this record in the future. Oh how I wish that I could produce the sort of journal entries penned by a character created by Oscar Wilde, who declares, "I never travel without my diary. One should always have something sensational to read in the train."

Journal entries can be discontinuous from day to day. Therefore, during one week a succession of topics can take up my interest, but during another week every entry may obsess over a single communication problem I am having with a relative. I can be motivated to write by a famous line of poetry—"Death is the mother of beauty"—that inexplicably infuriates me. I might compose a screed on the bollixed up billing of a CT scan. News of a friend's recurrence—from whom and when I received it, how it began to upset me, in what ways I might be able to help—means I need to express my grief.

During some treatments, I mock or whine or rant about my miseries, or lie to myself royally. At times, my journal revolves around visiting friends; at other times, it tackles the writing quandaries ensnaring me. Frequently, I make reading lists or lists of topics that intrigue me, or describe puzzling dreams so I can return to them at another writing session. Many authors have used their diaries as a painter would a sketchbook—trying out colors and shapes and designs, working out conceptual snags, finding the right perspective or tone. Virginia Woolf sought to keep her diary "so elastic that it will embrace anything," like "a deep old desk" in which "one flings a mass of odds & ends."

Free and compulsive writers alike must, of course, decide upon the implements, places, and timings of their sessions. Will you write with a pen or pencil in a spiral notebook, or on a keyboard with a screen? As many doctors say when patients confront impossibly difficult choices about treatment, "It's up to you!" For years, I could write only by hand with a number 2 pencil on yellow legal pads, and then I switched to blue pens and those black-and-white mottled notebooks. But later I started working on a typewriter with little jars of Wite-Out, and then at a computer from which I had to print out every afternoon; and now I use a laptop, printing out toward the end of multiple revisions on the screen. (Actually, I have never printed out my post-recurrence diary, which is very long, or my blogs, which are very short—I simply reread on the screen—but the chapters of this book had to be printed out repeatedly.)

Where will you write? During high school, I started out in crowded cafeterias, moved on to library carrels in college, graduated to a desk in my faculty office, settled down in the driver's seat of my car between endless chauffeuring stints for children, and ended up on the blue couch after surgery. At what time? When my kids were young, it depended on the babysitter's schedule, but now I find my most productive hours are from 10 a.m. till 2 p.m. There have been plenty of days when very little time can be carved out for writing, but I firmly believe that daily, habitual practice remains the most critical factor in sustaining writing.

So the most important question—deserving two paragraphs of its own—is how long and how often should you write? Although some teachers argue that beginners should write for 20 or 30 minutes every day, others believe that the goal should be 1,000 words (three or four printed pages) every day. This last would be an unrealistically high goal for me. Still, the key, I believe, is to write as much as possible. When I was leading a workshop of graduate students that we called TDF—The Dissertation Factory—our motto was "Place the seat of the pants on the seat of the chair." The point was not to let distractions or inhibitions stymie the writing process. The novelist Doris Lessing is typical in believing that "you only learn to be a better writer by actually writing." The punchline of the old joke asking "How do I get to Carnegie Hall?" pertains: "Practice, practice, practice."

Writing teachers unanimously agree that the more people write, the more fluent their writing becomes. This is why I used to advise my graduate students not to put off writing until they had completed their research. It is far better to engage in whatever reading needs to be done not before but while drafting and revising. If ice skaters or cellists or runners miss too many practice sessions, they lose muscle memory and stamina. I remember a time when a two-page letter of recommendation would take me a full day, and today I can churn one out in an hour—like an old sausage mill, my former collaborator and I joke. Diaries that pertain to the everyday occurrences of our lives draw our attention to the meaning of the everyday occurrences of our lives, so it makes sense to date entries. And, yes, take a holiday on weekends . . . unless the magnetic draw of your journal compels you back.

Whether you are a free or a compulsive writer, one reward of keeping a journal is lightening the load on others. Especially during the long haul of chronic disease, friends and family can tolerate hearing only so much and probably not much more. Who wants to be a bore, droning on about subjects that will inspire sadness or, worse, pity in people then made afraid to confide their own concerns, lest they seem trivial compared to yours? In dealing with depression after a breast cancer diagnosis, the memoirist Kathlyn Conway found that "Writing gave me the freedom to be honest in a way that was not always possible in conversation, where, I found, people sometimes cut me off or subtly let me know that they wanted to hear only a particular version of my experience."

But daily writing does more than provide an outlet for venting without self-censorship. Even when it tackles the miseries of treatment or the disease's progression, it can also become an escape hatch. Instead of obsessing over a scar, in my journal I find myself obsessing over words to convey what it looks like. Instead of worrying about my sense of inauthenticity in a wig, I find myself trying to capture that worry in language conveying my need not to be instantly identified as a cancer patient in every social event I encounter. (I'm wearing the wig I call Torian Gray in the author photo for this book.) In this regard, writing induces a posture of detachment or provides a counterirritant.

At the risk of stating the obvious, writing about cancer is not quite the same as having cancer. In the process of describing disease, we distance ourselves from it. Writing puts us at a remove from the phenomena being recorded (which is why so many movies about writing are so boring). While writing, I dwell not on the here and now but on a representation of the here and now—or some there and then—that resurrects itself with a new meaning or symmetry and a different vantage. Relating this logic about verbal representations to visual ones, the painter René Magritte famously inscribed a sentence over a realistic picture of a pipe he had painted: "Ceci n'est pas une pipe" (This is not a pipe). To understand his point, simply invert the title of Wallace Stevens's poem "Not Ideas about the Thing but the Thing Itself": writing, like painting, produces not the pipe itself, but ideas about the pipe. While writing, we become less sick or debilitated because we are conceptualizing how it feels or what it means to be sick or debilitated. The words "compose" and "composure"—when we are composing an essay—point toward this phenomenon.

Thus far, I have been assuming that cancer patients want or need to write about their disease. But as my reference above to "some there and then" indicates, writing about the past before diagnosis also meets a pressing need. The shock of mortality that illness triggers can flood patients not only with dread of the future but also with memories of the past. Only after a leukemia diagnosis did the prominent postcolonial thinker Edward Said feel impelled to recount his scholarship's origins in his formative years: "I found myself trying to make sense of my own life as its end seemed alarmingly nearer." After the physician-author Oliver Sacks discovered cancer in his liver, he found that working on his autobiography helped free him from obsessive worries.

The urgency of retrospection, stock-taking, looking back on good times, contending with old grievances can be overwhelming. When grueling treatments make it impossible for me to recognize my diminished self, it helps to recall pivotal moments before cancer when I took great pleasure in some small accomplishment in parenting or in pursuing my profession. In my diary, I can move forward into the past by considering the dismal mortifications and luscious pleasures of a youthful love affair, recollections of adolescence, and ambivalent early relationships with my parents. I can dwell on what I will miss most by dying. But, then again, I often use my diary to plan menus of meals that do and do not take place.

Venting and escaping, distracting oneself and stock-taking should not be undervalued; however, a diary also helps us understand and alter our condition. Journals can assist patients in talking with or back to physicians, nurses, and caregivers in a safe place that functions as a rehearsal space for subsequent real conversations that influence future decisions about treatment. Do I want to undergo radiation or surgery, or should I engage in watchful waiting? A list of pros and cons can clarify the issues and consequences at stake. It might be best to consult oneself on these complex matters before and while gaining the advice of medical authorities. In a journal, it is possible to work through difficult emotional reactions and find the right cadence to converse with and perhaps modify the behavior of negligent or overly assiduous caretakers, scared-away friends or ghoulish acquaintances, troubled parents and children.

If I know that I am going to record an event, like an upcoming and difficult conversation, I become more mindful about analyzing its subtleties while I engage in it. The very prospect of writing focuses my attention. And the daily rhythm of keeping a diary—which can be reread to remind us of our remote and recent past and to give us ideas about future writing possibilities—produces steadiness, acceptance, sometimes even euphoria. (Am I beginning to sound like a used-car salesman?) For some people, the process of writing delivers a newborn and stronger self into the world. The breast cancer activist Musa Mayer believes that "writing about my illness has provided for me a sort of armature upon which I can deposit, as a sculptor does bits of wet clay, the raw substance of memory and experience to form a new image, a new sense of who I am."

As in the act of sculpting clay or the performance of certain rituals, in the process of composition time can slow down and in an odd way stand still. When writing becomes a rite, it generates an absorbing form of concentration that is accompanied by the pleasures of zoning out and tuning in and turning on—with the added bonus of producing a durable text. Daily composition—on whatever subject takes our fancy—liberates patients from endemic feelings of helpless abjection. For people who have been forced to hand their bodies and their lives over to oncologists, radiologists, and surgeons, composition reinstates some control. On the page or screen, with words, we can recapture an elsewhere imperiled sense of freedom and autonomy. Even the deleterious side effects of cancer regimes can be circumvented by writing, for a journal can be picked up and put down, it may involve ten minutes or two hours, it can be sidelined during bouts of pain, and it need never see the light of day.

Indeed, the privacy of a diary is its greatest good; maintaining a diary can conserve discretion. Despite a culture addicted to tawdry self-display, quite a few cancer patients opt for reticence. Think of Rachel Carson, who kept her cancer a secret so that her ecological work in *Silent Spring* would not be dismissed as personally motivated; or the brilliant comic writer Nora Ephron, whose friends were shocked to learn after her death that she had been dealing with leukemia. My mentor, the literary critic and detective novelist Carolyn Heilbrun, never told me that in her young adulthood she had undergone a mastectomy; I learned about it in a biography published after her death. Since I have been very open about my disease, I did not fully understand this sort of secrecy until I read Henry James's novel *The Wings of the Dove*, in which every character wonders what exactly ails dying Milly Theale.

James's heroine clings to her privacy, refusing to communicate her symptoms—and why not, James makes us realize. Rather than being bowed down by the specificity of her complaints, the burden of other people's commiserations, the demeaning details of a sickness's progression, or a physician's guess at its projected progression, Milly Theale decides to be active "as if it were in her power to live":

"she favoured every idea, but most of all the idea that she herself was to go on as if nothing were the matter." With dignity and courage, she makes her remaining days on earth an extension of her life, not the prelude to her death. All of which is a roundabout way of honoring private patients who can use their journals in defense of their "ferocity of modesty"—a wonderful James phrase. And of course there are pragmatic reasons to keep writing private. No need to deal with rejection letters from publishers, criticism from editors, obtuse reviewers, or sarcastic readers. Since there are many ways to hide a diary, the vexed problem of self-exposure need not be an impediment.

So how to begin? The best response to this question I have ever heard or read arrives in Anne Lamott's account of her 10-year-old brother "trying to get a report on birds written that he'd had three months to write, which was due the next day." Lamott tells this story because it captures "the tremendous sense of being overwhelmed" that her students experience. I always quoted it in my writing courses because my students also suffered from a sense of being overwhelmed, and so here it is:

> We were out at our family cabin in Bolinas, and he was at the kitchen table close to tears, surrounded by binder paper and pencils and unopened books on birds, immobilized by the hugeness of the task ahead. Then my father sat down beside him, put his arm around my brother's shoulder, and said, "Bird by bird, buddy. Just take it bird by bird."

I often tell myself, "Susan, just take it bird by bird." But sometimes I want a little inspiration to find trenchant or evocative ways of recording my thoughts and feelings. Then I reach for the stars—

the illustrious authors whose works provide a model for all sorts of writing strategies—and take them one by one.

What we read fuels what we write. Among the most notable of cancer diarists, Fanny Burney, Alice James, and Audre Lorde produced prose that employs some of the techniques that patient-writers can use to strengthen our work. If we study their productions, we can aspire to gain the immediacy they achieved in their depictions of their struggles with illness. That all of them confronted breast cancer illustrates the disproportionate amount of writing about this particular form of the disease.

Despite the commonality of their subject, their works exhibit strikingly different strengths, for Fanny Burney excels in characterization and plotting, Alice James in an exceptionally eccentric voice, Audre Lorde in polemical argumentation. Taken together, they suggest that a powerful letter or diary entry depends on the same elements usually associated with fiction: character, plot, point of view, setting, and dialogue interspersed with description. Keeping these elements in mind can make us more effective writers.

Fanny Burney's March 22, 1812, letter to her sister describes a mastectomy undertaken in a period before anesthetics and antisepsis. Of course the pain she recounts during the cutting of her breast remains indelibly shocking, but what makes the account leading up to the operation vivid are the characters she brings to life. First, there is her beloved husband, a major wuss. After a consultation with a celebrated surgeon, Burney's husband never appears to tell her what the conversation revealed. Instead, M. d'A. (as she calls him) hides out. His nonappearance after the doctor's departure greatly alarms her and she begs him to return to her company, which he does:

> He, also, sought then to tranquilize me—but in words only; his looks were shocking! his features, his whole face displayed the bitterest woe. I had not, therefore, much difficulty in telling myself what he endeavored not to tell me—that a small operation would be necessary to avert evil consequences!

Concern over her "too sympathizing partner" subsequently causes the frightened Fanny to shield her husband not only from the sight of the operation but even beforehand from knowledge of when it will occur. Through her portrait of his character, Fanny Burney illuminates the caregiving that cancer patients sometimes need to provide their caregivers.

When Burney finally receives the "summons to execution," a phrase that conveys her horror of her "doom," she reads the letter conveying information on the doctors' proposed date of arrival, knowing that she has to disguise her reaction from her husband:

> I affected to be long reading the note, to gain time for forming some plan, & such was my terror of involving M. d'A. in the unavailing wretchedness of witnessing what I must go through, that it conquered every other, & gave me the force to act as if I were directing some third person.

Not at all sardonic about her husband's heightened sensibilities, Burney seems instead rather proud of them and protective of him. Curiously, his weakness strengthens her. And he appears infinitely grateful to be kept at some remove from the surgical horrors she watched through a cloth placed on her face.

Burney's lengthy letter captures the medical mores of the early nineteenth century, which in some regards do not seem far removed from the customs of today: the jockeying between specialists, the tricky etiquette involved in getting a second opinion, the arrogance of physicians who dictate the timing of events at their own convenience and thereby instigate the "dreadful interval" of "never-ending" hours of waiting until Burney becomes "stupid—torpid, without sentiment or consciousness." Again, the characters dramatize these issues. The celebrated doctor M. Dubois, for instance, produces a "long & unintelligible harangue," acts as "commander in chief" as he issues "his commands *en militaire*," and uses his imperious finger to orchestrate the other physicians as they make the necessary incisions.

But her (and my) favorite doctor is the lugubrious M. Larrey, whose genius in the medical profession is matched only by "an ignorance of the world & its usages that induces a *naïveté* that leads those who do not see him thoroughly to think him not alone simple, but weak": "his attention & thoughts having exclusively turned one way, he is hardly awake any other." A physician who gloomily suffers along with his patients, M. Larrey often visits Burney, but pronounces nothing and appears "always melancholy."

All the coming-and-going characters and all the trepidation and waiting expressed in Fanny Burney's letter build to the climactic mastectomy scene that serves as the culmination of her plot. She slows down the pace of narration when "7 men in black" enter her room, and then describes a multitude of very specific details: the cambric handkerchief spread upon her face, the glitter of polished steel, the forefinger of M. Dubois outlining "a straight line from top to bottom of the breast, secondly a cross, & thirdly a circle," the plunging steel "cutting through veins—arteries—flesh—nerves," the painful wound "like a mass of minute but sharp & forked poniards" (daggers), the instrument "cutting against the grain . . . while the flesh resisted in a manner so forcibly as to oppose & tire the hand of the operator, who was forced to change from the right to the left," the interminable scraping. So sustained is the scene that it is surprising to read toward the end of this account that the operation lasted 20 minutes. Without anesthesia and punctuated by her recurrent loss of consciousness, those 20 minutes must have felt like 20 hours, or so her genius makes us feel. Though I have been known to rant against contemporary medical technologies, Fanny Burney makes me grateful for them.

Burney's example suggests that we might profitably engage in character sketches of ourselves and of the caregivers and doctors with whom we interact by conveying scenes of our relationships with them. In her pages, we encounter few heroes or villains, but many personalities with subtly delineated temperaments. She also reminds us of the efficacy of letters. Many people compose their journals as a succession of letters to themselves or to an ideal reader or directly to their diaries. In my experience unsent letters can be more cathartic than sent letters, since all the anger and hurt or guilt and shame I might feel in a particular situation with a specific person gets distilled without the need of holding back to spare that person's feelings. Since Burney composed this particular letter for her sister and knew that it would be shown to Esther's circle, throughout she assures her readers that she survived with the strength to tell the tale well.

Whereas Burney excels in characterization and the piling up of very specific, tactile details, Alice James achieves an idiosyncratic voice in her diary when she welcomes cancer as her heart's desire, a cherished destiny. In part, her strange elation arose because she had suffered from a host of mysterious symptoms—cardiac attacks, fainting spells, headache, paralyzed legs, gout—for two decades before she received the cancer diagnosis in May 1891. Alice James would die the next year at the age of 44. Her entry on discovering the breast cancer begins with eerie jubilation: "To him who waits, all things come!" Then, fully aware of the oddity of her reaction, she explains why cancer represents the fulfillment of her aspirations:

> Ever since I have been ill, I have longed and longed for some palpable disease, no matter how conventionally dreadful a label it might have, but I was always driven back to stagger alone under the monstrous mass of subjective sensations, which that sympathetic being "the medical man" had no higher inspiration than to assure me I was personally responsible for, washing his hands of me with a graceful complacency under my very nose.

Resentful that her doctors dismissed her ills as psychosomatic, blamed her for them, and treated her as if she were mentally defective, she feels relief when the physician Sir Andrew Clark "endowed" her "not only with cardiac complications" but also with the knowledge that the "lump" in her breast is a tumor, and "that nothing can be done for me but to alleviate pain, that it is only a question of time, etc." Yet elation at the cancer diagnosis goes beyond relief at finding a physiological cause of her suffering. When added to her other miseries, the diagnosis "ought to satisfy the most inflated pathologic vanity." Alice James cannot take pride in her accomplishments in the world, so she determines perversely to take pride in her multiple ailments. Celebrating her brother Henry's published novels that year and the appearance of her brother William's massive book on psychology, she finds it "not a bad show for one family!" and then adds mordantly, "especially if I get myself dead, the hardest job of all."

Surely Alice James knew that her determination to get herself dead was not a normal or healthy response, but she insists on flouting conventional judgment. She becomes disappointed with the tumor when she realizes that it may take longer to kill her than she first expected. After being told she might live some months, she deadpans, "This is a strain." She savors the absurdities she encounters through illness. To the cancer, for instance, she attributes the deepening of her relationship with her companion, Katharine Loring: "As the ugliest things go to the making of the fairest, it is not wonderful that this unholy granite substance in my breast should be the soil propitious for the perfect flowering of Katharine's unexampled genius for friendship and devotion."

One of Alice James's favorite pastimes involves her watching Katharine reduce prominent British doctors to "impotent paralysis." Like Sir Andrew, "they are all terrible, with that globular manner, talking by the hour without *saying* anything, while the longing pallid victim stretches out a sickly tendril, hoping for some excrescence, a human wart, to catch on to, but it vainly slips off the polished surface, as comforting and nourishing as that of a billiard ball." What a hilarious send-up of medical professionalism! The word "globular" brilliantly prepares for the avuncular polish of the "billiard ball" physicians.

Valuing not the extension of her life but the maintenance of her self-respect through mockery and self-mockery, Alice James eventually finds her "long slow dying . . . disappointingly free from excitements." She therefore focuses on her integrity, the "satisfaction in feeling as much myself as ever, perhaps simply a more concentrated essence in this curtailment." Shocked when a visitor tells her that she will live "a good bit still," she finds the thought "*inconvenient*," but then is gladdened. For the visitor has offered her the opportunity "to test the sincerity of my mortuary inclinations": "I have always *thought* that I wanted to die, but I felt quite uncertain as to what my muscular demonstrations might be at the moment of transition, for I occasionally have a quiver as of an expected dentistical wrench when I fancy the actual moment." Being annoyed with her visitor's optimism assures her that she will "be able to maintain a calm befitting so sublimated a spirit!" And then in defense of her "mortuary inclinations," she characteristically warns herself, "'twould be such a bore to be perturbed."

Alice James dictated to her companion Katharine Loring the final sentences about pain grinding her down, when she almost asked for "K.'s lethal dose," but refrained from "such unaccustomed ways." Instead of resorting to suicide, she contrasts physical pain to worse torments: "physical pain however great ends in itself and falls away like dry husks from the mind, whilst moral discords and nervous horrors sear the soul." Having mastered hypnosis, Katharine has these mental discords and horrors so "completely under the control of her rhythmic hand" that Alice need no longer dread them.

Paradoxical to the end, though, she considers the consolation of hypnosis and then rejects it, because it distracts her from what she wants to attend: her mortuary consciousness. First she recalls "the wonderful moment when I felt myself floated for the first time into the deep sea of divine *cessation*, and saw all the dear old mysteries and miracles vanish into vapour!" Immediately afterward, she counts herself fortunate that this experience has not been repeated, because "it might become a seduction." Stoical, Alice James watches her own dying with ironic detachment.

The example of Alice James suggests that the old writing adage "Show, don't tell" ain't necessarily so. With very few dramatic scenes, she nevertheless proves that powerful prose springs out of integrity to the self, even and perhaps especially when it is achieved by abrogating generally accepted values, thereby risking the possibility of shocking readers. Her achievement puts me in mind of Anatole Broyard's comment about the most efficacious response to disease: "I would advise every sick person to evolve a style or develop a voice for his or her illness." The reasoning behind his remark relates to Alice James's sense of her doctors as polished billiard balls. The impersonality of medical personnel—especially when their contact is so physically intimate—can deprive patients of a sense of humanity, even as the generic role of patient can erode a sense of individuality.

To craft an assertively individualistic voice of one's own, it is easiest to write in the first person. But sometimes it helps to experiment with switching tones: to try out, for example, Alice James's sardonic intonation or the melodramatic register of a soap opera character or the terse words of a hard-boiled detective. That Alice James when incapacitated asked her companion to record her sentences reminds me that today all sorts of dictation devices are available for those who cannot physically use a keyboard or a pen.

Alice James's acerbic eccentricity contrasts sharply with Audre Lorde's fervent insistence on helping other women profit from her experiences. Yet Lorde also crafted a highly individuated voice. Since she was a poet before she was a cancer patient, it is hardly surprising that *The Cancer Journals* is studded with metaphors, images, and analogies that capture her affiliations as a black lesbian activist. The book consists of two sorts of discourses: an introduction and three essays that are spliced with italicized entries from a journal started six months after Audre Lorde's mastectomy. Imbued with her determination to convert pain and fear into empowering forms of knowledge, *The Cancer Journals* was published in 1980, at the apex of the second wave of feminism.

In the first reprinted journal entry, Lorde describes pain that "*fills me like a puspocket and every touch threatens to breach the taut membrane that keeps it from flowing through and poisoning my whole existence. Sometimes despair sweeps across my consciousness like luna winds across a barren moonscape. Ironshod horses range back and forth over every nerve.*" Startling images are juxtaposed here without any effort at coherence in order to capture feelings difficult to communicate.

In her retrospective, essayistic prose (without italics), she uses more sustained images. About a biopsy proving that she has cancer, for instance, Lorde records a number of different mental responses that together constitute "a concert of voices from inside myself, all with something slightly different to say, all of which were quite insistent and none of which would let me rest." After the mastectomy, her "breast which was no longer there would hurt as if it were being squeezed in a vise. That was perhaps the worst pain of all, because it would come with a full complement of horror that I was to be forever reminded of my loss by suffering in a part of me which was no longer there."

Throughout *The Cancer Journals*, Lorde creates hospital scenes that fill her with dread or sorrow. After she loses sight of her partner Frances's face "like a great sunflower in the sky," Lorde records the trip to the operating room:

> There is the horror of those flashing lights passing over my face, and the clanging of disemboweled noises that have no context nor relationship to me except they assault me. There is the dispatch with which I have ceased being a person who is

myself and become a thing upon a Guerney cart to be delivered
up to Moloch, a dark living sacrifice in the white place.

When a few days later a "kindly woman from Reach for Recovery"
visits Lorde's room, takes off her jacket, and displays her chest in
a sweater to prove that a prosthesis effectively hides the loss of a
breast, Lorde politely admits that she cannot "tell which is which."
However, she then adds,

> In her tight foundation garment and stiff, up-lifting bra, both
> breasts looked equally unreal to me. But then I've always been
> a connoisseur of women's breasts, and never overly fond of stiff
> uplifts. I looked away, thinking, "I wonder if there are any
> black lesbian feminists in Reach for Recovery?"

Finally alone, Lorde stands before a mirror and stuffs the "gro-
tesquely pale" lamb's wool into her bra, finds it even more alienating than her flat chest, and returns to bed to cry herself to sleep.

Audre Lorde bristles at the injunction to use a prosthesis,
because "*it feels like a lie more than a costume.*" She is particularly
enraged at "a charmingly bright and steady" nurse who urged her
"to wear something, at least when you come in [to see the doctor].
Otherwise it's bad for the morale of the office." To defend her decision not to hide "behind a pathetic puff of lambswool which has
no relationship nor likeness" to her own breasts, Lorde chooses a
telling analogy:

> When Moishe Dayan, the Prime Minister of Israel, stands
> up in front of parliament or on TV with an eyepatch over his
> empty eye socket, nobody tells him to go get a glass eye, or

that he is bad for the morale of the office. The world sees him as a warrior with an honorable wound, and a loss of a piece of himself which he has marked, and mourned, and moved beyond. And if you have trouble dealing with Moishe Dayan's empty eye socket, everyone recognizes that it is your problem to solve, not his.

Lorde wants her loss to be "an honorable reminder" that she is "a casualty in the cosmic war against radiation, animal fat, air pollution, McDonald's hamburgers and Red Dye No. 2," and that "the fight is still going on, and I am still a part of it."

Already out of the closet as a lesbian, Lorde decides to be out as a cancer patient as well. She associates the social pressure to wear a prosthesis with a culture that wants to silence and separate women: "what would happen if an army of one-breasted women descended upon Congress and demanded that the use of carcinogenic, fat-stored hormones in beef-feed be outlawed?" *The Cancer Journals* ends with a scathing attack on the American Cancer Society for failing to deal with prevention. During a period of time when some implants were carcinogenic, she lambastes a cosmetic surgery industry that encourages a woman to get "a sack of silicone implanted under her skin" with the argument that "a woman may well be more likely to die from another cancer, but without that implant . . . she is not 'feminine.'"

Even in the italicized journal entries composed directly after her surgery, Lorde struggles against despair by transforming an anguished cry into language that empowers her to stand up for her convictions. So, in a diary entry placed near the close of her book, she wants to say that "*I'd give anything not to have cancer,*" but she immediately lists what she would *not* in fact give up: she would not renounce her life, or her partner, or her poetry, or her eyes, or her arms. And this realization allows her to acknowledge that the sexual pleasure connected with her right breast—which she had feared losing—can never be lost, because it resides within her and because "I can attach it anywhere I want to." Cancer, neither a gift nor an opportunity, cannot turn her into a victim. She ends her book with the sentence "I would never have chosen this path, but I am very glad to be who I am, here."

The uses to which the painter Hollis Sigler put Audre Lorde's words demonstrate the unpredictable ways in which diaries generate diaries. In *Hollis Sigler's Breast Cancer Journal*, a series of paintings in storybook colors illuminate the artist's response to a disease that became metastatic. On the frames and also in the spacers between the paper and the glass of framed drawings, Sigler inscribed her outrage about the facts of the epidemic as well as excerpts from Lorde's *Cancer Journals* and her own diaries.

Sigler's paintings brood over the loneliness of cancer—rarely do they show human figures—and the losses of disease: we see shattered mirrors, tattered dresses, empty rooms, barren trees, wind- and firestorms threatening a home. A shocking lack of control is depicted as food and silverware unexpectedly fly up off a table. The image reminds me of Dr. Benedict B. Benigno's belief that "if life is a banquet, then cancer takes away the knife and fork and pulls the chair out from under us." Yet the most disturbing pictures blaze with a joyful vibrancy, a childlike spontaneity transmitted by a faux naïve style. The brightly patterned images glow with the artist's love of the life she knows she will soon have to leave.

❊

The gritty immediacy of Lorde's italicized journal entries proves that one need not and perhaps ought not always edit and revise. However, these fragmented quotations appear within an introduction and three essays that exhibit the polish of retrospective, finished prose. Focused and structured, *The Cancer Journals* departs from the daily diary form to deliver the sort of lesson implicit in the subtitle of its last chapter, "Power vs. Prosthesis": a case against padding and reconstructive surgery. Such a rubric hints at an argument expounded through a series of autobiographical accounts, critiques of hospital protocols, and quotations from medical experts. Together, the evidence mounts to clarify a thesis that may sound anachronistic in today's world of successful breast reconstructions, but that remains rhetorically powerful.

Focus and structure do not pertain to the capacious diary and therefore are best left to the next chapter about published work and to the final chapter about posted blogs. However, other aspects of revision do relate to journal entries and to the essays or blogs that may derive from them, and so they can be raised here, if only in a brief digression.

Some proponents of free writing dismiss revision, fearing that worries about grammar and style will discourage people by reminding them of the mistakes they might make. (If such discussions inhibit you, skip the next few pages.) Should you be using a diary entry as a draft for work you want to share, however, you may find revising a supreme source of pleasure, as I do because it leads me to become clearer about my intentions. And of course if you aim to polish your freewriting for wider circulation, you will want to ensure that it is grammatical. A classic on proper usage—William Strunk and E. B. White's *Elements of Style*—admits that excellent writers sometimes disregard grammar, but adds a caution: "Unless he is certain of doing well," the writer "will probably do best to follow the rules." No less an authority than Stephen King agrees, and in *On Writing* he recommends *Warriner's English Grammar and Composition* to those in need of help. Today there are numerous online sites—like OWL—to help with grammar and syntax.

Tangled in a morass of sentences, I continue to make every grammatical error that my freshmen used to make (and so do many seasoned writers). In a hilarious send-up called "How to Write a Sentence"—focusing on sentences as "the building blobs of a paragraph"—James Thomas chuckles over our gaffes: "Mistakes are whom makes us what we are." Grammatical glitches remain a lifelong challenge for many. Months after my husband first laughed at the inscription in the lobby of the Simon Cancer Center—"WE, WHO EXPERIENCE CANCER, THANK MARVIN AND BREN SIMON"—I could not untangle his logic. "A restrictive modifier cannot have a comma," Don explained. "A nonrestrictive modifier can be taken out of the sentence and its fundamental meaning will not change." Still I remained dubious of my understanding (and I had at that point been teaching English for decades).

A year later, I stood in the lobby and a lightbulb went on: those people who have experienced cancer are thanking the Simons. The commas had to go! (We emailed my oncologist, who emailed a hospital administrator who—you guessed it—did nothing at all.) One need not know grammatical terms—"a nonrestrictive modifier"— to develop a good ear or eye that hears or sees "the building blobs" that need to be changed.

Teachers of writing distinguish grammatical errors from stylistic problems that can become just as absorbing. Stephen King offers a funny example of the passive voice: "My first kiss will always be recalled by me as how my romance with Shayna was begun." The polemicist Christopher Hitchens believed that the best advice he received was to write "more like the way you talk." But he, too, cautioned against stylistic howlers, especially poor word placement: "Don't say that as a boy your grandmother used to read to you, unless at that stage of her life she really *was* a boy, in which case you have probably thrown away a better intro." All advisors tell writers to rework weak verbs (versions of "is") and to avoid silly adverbs ("shockingly") and clichés ("like the plague"), word repetition and wordiness, vague generalizations, bumpy transitions, paragraphs that are a page long, and a vocabulary that is either too limited or sounds pretentious. Stephen King's example of this last trap—"John stopped long enough to perform an act of excretion"—makes me wish I had had his book when I was putting together handouts for my freshmen.

Consider all the ways in which "John stopped long enough to perform an act of excretion" could be changed. Revision functions as a godsend when you get stuck in drafting. Actually, any and all switching of gears works: typing what is handwritten, changing the font or the spacing, printing out and rereading, reading aloud. Revision keeps you focused on the work at hand. It might involve playing around with paragraphs—changing their order, moving the conclusion to the introduction—or noting and fixing the monotony of a succession of sentences with the exact same syntax or checking the obsessive repetition of one word.

But revision can also become self-subverting. The most dysfunctional academic writer I ever knew, and there have been quite a few, saved every draft on her computer as a new file. So, for example, if she fixed too many sentences beginning with present participles ("ing" verbal forms), she saved that as file Y. If she later revised file Y so as to remove the word "only," which recurred too often, she saved it as file W. Save your work, but not all of your work, or you will drive yourself crazy.

John's stopping to perform an act of excretion also reminds me that medical language—often so incomprehensible or stilted in its specialized jargon—offers patients a unique opportunity to translate ugly-sounding Latin and Greek terms into visceral descriptions of what they mean to the person that they have labeled. The arcane language of specialists often proves trying for patients who have no idea what "creatinine" or "platelets," "ecog status" or "neutrophil counts" really mean or how those terms may impinge on their lives.

In a novel titled *The Sickness*, by the Venezuelan writer Alberto Barrera Tyszka, a physician whose father is dying of lung cancer "finds the clinical terms unbearable," forming "part of a pretentious, useless dictionary":

> neoplasty exeresis staphylococcal empyema
> pleural empyema anastomosis ileocolostomy
> biopsy haemostasis prosthesis laparatomy
> ischemia lithiasis.

For years, I was stymied by the word "anastomosis": it stood in the way of my understanding what had happened within my body. Just as incomprehensible are the acronyms resounding in hospital halls—PIC, BRCA, PSA, NPO, PEG, NG, PTN, PK, HER2, DCIS, LCIS—that need to be decoded, or they degenerate into an unpalatable alphabet soup.

Too many medical terms seem to blame patients—who have "relapsed" or become "platinum resistant," or whose margins or scans are "not clean," or who are said to have "failed a treatment" when the treatment has really failed them. Or some doctors' phrases mask brutal realities with euphemisms about, say, "minimal or acceptable side effects." To unmask those realities, Dr. Susan Love translated surgery, radiation, and chemotherapy into "slash, burn, and poison." Patients, too, have created a number of coinages, such as "scanxiety" (fearful anticipation of a scan) and "chemoflage" (cheerful misinformation in chemotherapy booklets). Fulminating against the term "survivor," one reader of my essays in the *New York Times* defined herself as "PHD" (Patient Hasn't Died), another as "a chemosapien" (a being perpetually on chemo).

In an article encouraging linguistic exuberance, the witty queer theorist Eve Kosofsky Sedgwick recommended self-defining acronyms like BBP (Bald Barfing Person) and WAPHMO (Woman About to Go Postal at HMO). She then confided that she personally had alternated between PSHIFTY (Person Still Hanging in Fine Thank You) and QIBIFA (Quite Ill But, Inexplicably, Fat Anyway) until she settled on "undead." To describe herself when she would no longer qualify to be numbered among the undead, Sedgwick decided on "differently extant."

This last formation especially helps me come to terms with my future condition. For those of us writing about living with the dysfunctional body, though, the issue of lexicon and tone will remain dicey. Sometimes I try out the in-your-face vulgarity of street talk, sometimes the circumlocutions of polite society, sometimes the potty mouth of kindergartners, for our hearing changes as we evolve in our reading, which remains the single most formative influence on our writing.

Like Fanny Burney and Alice James, Audre Lorde shared her writing about cancer with friends; unlike them, she lived to see it published. I expect to keep my diary private simply because that way I can be totally honest in it. So it is hidden on my computer within an oddly named folder that none of my survivors would think to scrutinize. Probably I will delete it before my death. Yet I continue to use it not only to record and reflect on my life but also to try out various strategies: a character sketch, a socially unsanctioned reaction, a potent analogy. As the first sentence of this chapter demonstrates, I often try to imitate or invoke the style of admired novelists, paying particular attention to the shape of their sentences: the equanimity and balance of Jane Austen's phrases, the curt reportage of a series of short Ernest Hemingway statements, the remarkably fluid stream of consciousness pioneered by Virginia Woolf. A tried-and-true method of learning how to write, imitation can propel all sorts of composition ventures. What would Dr. Seuss or, for that matter, Stephen King produce in response to one of the writing prompts suggested earlier? (That's an assignment it might be fun to take on.)

In my diary, I have participated in a phenomenon that has only recently become apparent to me: writing at the end of life to and for survivors. Because dealing with cancer generally accords people the time necessary to be aware of death's approach, we can use that awareness to make preparations, say goodbye, or advocate for various causes.

Since diagnosis, I have composed a series of letters to be given to my children, my stepchildren, and their children after my death. In them, I recount jokes, recall musical or sports performances during their school years, thank them for material and nonmaterial gifts, characterize their temperaments at birth or what I made of them when I first met them, embarrass them with stories about gaffes they and I have committed, regale them with cooking adventures and vacation misadventures, and remind them of celebrations we relished together. Although I periodically return to thicken these letters, at some point I may print them and put them in addressed envelopes. Twenty-nine-year-old Brittany Maynard used her remaining time with a terminal brain cancer to recount her story on the Internet in an effort to persuade Americans to extend Oregon's

Death with Dignity Act to other states: she posted notes and photos as well as a deadline for her own planned demise.

*The Last Lecture* by Randy Pausch, a popular Web video and best-selling book, exemplifies the effort to create a posthumous voice. In September 2007, Professor Pausch delivered a spirited lecture on the cognitive dissonance between his physical well-being and the diagnosis he was facing of a pancreatic cancer that would end up killing him in July 2008. He described his childhood dreams and his career in computer science, sang "Happy Birthday" to his wife, and used a PowerPoint slide to list the heartfelt but, to some, treacly life lessons he learned such as "Don't complain, just work harder" and "Find the best in everyone." Pausch concluded his lecture by admitting that his target audience consisted not of the people in the auditorium but of his children in their future without him.

According to the constitutionally satiric Christopher Hitchens, Pausch's sentiment—"so sugary that you need an insulin shot to withstand it"—and the mugging in front of a captive audience proved that "as the populations of Tumortown and Wellville continue to swell and to interact, there's a growing need for ground rules that prevent us from inflicting ourselves upon one another." Yet as Hitchens himself was dying from esophageal cancer, he continued to record his ongoing intellectual feuds, confident that they would be published posthumously, as they were in the book *Mortality*.

The self-obituary, a genre with quite a few how-to-do-it websites, seems to be coming into its own these days. In my hometown newspaper, a lengthy and laudatory obituary of a colleague persuaded a member of my cancer support group that this man must have been especially cherished. I did not have the heart to tell her that he had composed it himself. On the other hand, when my friend Pep's self-obit appeared in the local paper, I felt tears welling in my eyes: it was as if I heard his jokey, self-deprecating voice from beyond the grave. After a recurrence of endometrial cancer, the Seattle-based author and editor Jane Catherine Lotter posted a self-obit that went viral. Like Pep's, hers did not pretend to be authored by anyone other than herself. In it she recalled the high points of her education and career because she wanted to be "joyful about having a full life," rather than "sad about having to die." She closed with thanks for her family and ended with "Beautiful day, happy to have been here."

It is a much more gracious and generous piece of writing than an experiment I once wrote but never sent out for publication. After learning that two sisters had quarreled over what should and what should not be put into a third sister's obituary, I drafted a piece I called "Obitchuary" in which I annotated a boilerplate version of my obituary using the "track changes" function in Word. Next to the text, a series of marginal comments quibbled with the canned obit by voicing what any standard obituary leaves out: the messiness and confusion, the baser motives and ignoble emotions behind glib sentences about achievements and affiliations. If ever there were a therapeutic writing assignment, this was that.

Professional writers love talking about the horrors inflicted on them by their writing regimes: the torments of the blank page, the loneliness of isolation from the world, the Gobi Desert of slogging through the middle of a piece, the lacerating doubts about revision, and the postpartum depression after publication. Franz Kafka—famous for his scenes of irrationally inflicted torture—did write that "Writing is a sweet, wonderful reward," a sentiment much reproduced in Internet collections of quotes. However, he actually followed that claim by asking "but for what?" His answer: "it is the reward for serving the devil"! Allegiance to the devil's party has tempted quite a few writers to risk munching on the tempting fruits of knowledge.

Yet some prominent authors have extolled the benevolent pleasures of composition. The often-tormented Truman Capote said, "To me, the greatest pleasure of writing is not what it's about, but the music the words make." E. L. Doctorow felt that "Writing is an exploration. You start out from nothing and learn as you go." And Joyce Carol Oates believes that "The journal is the ideal place of refuge for the inner self because it constitutes a counterworld: a world to balance the other."

To my mind, Annie Dillard provides the clearest insight on the sovereignty of the writing life: "It is life at its most free, if you are fortunate enough to be able to try it, because you select your materials, invent your task, and pace yourself." She realizes that "The obverse of this freedom, of course, is that your work is so meaningless, so fully for yourself alone, and so worthless to the world, that no one except you cares whether you do it well, or ever." Many an author has taken that caveat as yet another liberty. Dillard also offers an imaginative route that may be easier for cancer patients than other would-be writers to follow: "Write as if you were dying. At the same time, assume you write for an audience consisting solely of terminal patients. That is, after all, the case. What would you begin writing if you knew you would die soon? What could you say to a dying person that would not enrage by its triviality?"

Too many books about the writing process are chockablock with patronizing rules, cajoling pleas, stern injunctions, and cute tips about how to stop procrastinating and get down to business. If I were to make one last recommendation, it would be to share any work you want to make public by signing up for a class or a conference or by participating in a small writing group whose members can serve as your first audience. Or do as I do, and exploit the good nature of your partner and friends. Especially if you hope to post or publish, it helps to have real readers, and before that—in the process of revision—to imagine your readers as specific people you know personally *and* as specific people you do not know personally. Should your envisioned audience consist of your baseball buddies and Mel Brooks or the Dalai Lama and your book club, you will have to devise strategies that draw them all into the scenario you are presenting.

But we have had more than enough of prescriptions. If you don't feel like writing, you might want to sample the outpouring of personal essays, memoirs, stories, novels, photographs, paintings, films, and television series that have been produced about living or dying with cancer. Or if you have already begun writing, one of these may serve in a mysterious way as a muse for your future work.

Chapter 2

# Impatient Memoirs

WHEN I WAS MOST incapacitated by treatment, the only activity that could pry me out of self-absorption was reading every cancer memoir I could get hold of—some produced by major publishing houses, some self-published. They proved the validity of an adage attributed to C. S. Lewis: "We read to know we are not alone." While immersed in the accounts of people confronting problems like mine, I feel less aberrant.

Because of their portability, books rescue me from the perpetual rounds of car trips, waiting rooms, and hospital stays. With my eyes glued to the page or screen, bleak settings fade into the background as I am conveyed into other worlds to connect with people who become my intimates. Alone even in a crowd and yet receiving communications from a dead or living author, I find in reading what Marcel Proust called "friendship brought back to its first purity," for there is no regret or fear about letting these friends down or displeasing them. Books do not care who is reading them, Allan Bennett reminds us in *The Uncommon Reader*. Indifferent to interruption and promiscuity, they can be put down, resumed, or abandoned for another after the blood draw or the taking of vitals. Far from being possessive, books lead the way to other books. In a book about a range of books that Will Schwalbe shared and discussed with his mother during her two-year struggle with pancreatic cancer, he found that "reading isn't the opposite of doing; it's the opposite of dying."

Although we also write to know we are not alone, the motivation of authors publishing books about their disease often goes beyond that incentive. Many memoir writers—distraught or incensed by the effects of cancer, by medical approaches to it, or by public understanding of it—broadcast their words to right such wrongs. In this regard, the authors of cancer memoirs have a surprisingly long lineage, dating back to ancient times. They resemble not the patient Job of legendary fame but the impatient Job who rails against the injustice of his miseries in the long complaints included in the biblical book named for him.

Stricken with loathsome sores from head to toe, Job gains in stature as he tenaciously laments his disease: "I loathe my life; / I will give free utterance to my complaint; / I will speak in the bitterness of my soul" (10:1). He bears witness to his suffering and his innocence with steadfast integrity, resisting the voices of those friends who view his illness as a just punishment or a learning experience. Surely, his smug advisors reason, Job must have been wicked to receive such pain. He must have smoked, refrained from exercise, consumed red meat, stressed out, repressed his anger, or, as Job's counselors explicitly claim, transgressed and sinned. Much to the surprise of most readers, at the end of the tale God rebukes them and affirms the righteousness of Job's honest expressions of anguish.

At the peak of his distress, Job utters a plea that illuminates the motives of patients and caregivers who publish memoirs about cancer:

O that my words were written down!
O that they were inscribed in a book!

O that with an iron pen and with lead
    they were engraved on a rock forever! (19:23–24)

The permanence of writing—inscribed in a book, engraved on a rock—would have solaced Job, lending him faith that a description of his hardships and a vindication of his character might survive his death. And we, reading his words in the Bible, realize that his wish has been granted.

Not all late twentieth- and early twenty-first-century accounts by patients are personal, but even when they eschew the personal they participate in Job's righteous effort to justify himself and his view of his situation. Susan Sontag's *Illness as Metaphor* was published two years after she was diagnosed with breast cancer, which she never mentions. Instead she targets the idea that "Patients who are instructed that they have, unwittingly, caused their disease are also being made to feel that they have deserved it." According to Sontag, literature and film and all sorts of scientific discourses promulgate damaging attitudes toward cancer. To her mind, the villains are the metaphors that cluster around these ailments—associations that continue to accrue when, for instance, politicians liken terrorist organizations to cancer cells.

Sontag attacked two pernicious notions prevalent in her time: that cancer is triggered by repressed anger and that it therefore should be blamed on the cancerous. Thanks in part to her book, we have moved beyond the period when patients were reduced to shameful silence. "My point," Sontag explains early on, "is that illness is *not* a metaphor, and that the most truthful way of regarding illness—and the healthiest way of being ill—is one purified of, most resistant to, metaphorical thinking."

Like Sontag, Stephen Jay Gould used his expertise to transform how we think about cancer. Gould began his 1985 essay "The Median

Isn't the Message" with his doctor telling him to abstain from reading scientific studies of abdominal mesothelioma, an incurable disease "with a median mortality of only eight months after discovery." An evolutionary biologist, he rejected this advice and employed his knowledge of statistics to counter the widespread anxiety of cancer patients about their chances of surviving.

Gould based his redefinition of what the median means on an assumption shared by evolutionary biologists: namely, "that variation itself is nature's only irreducible essence." The median isn't the message, because the variation is. Placing himself amid the variations— in part because his disease had been recognized at a relatively early stage—Gould noticed that graphs of the distribution of variations were right-skewed. The extended and right-skewed "tail" extended out for years beyond the eight-month median. "I saw no reason why I shouldn't be in that small tail, and I breathed a very long sigh of relief." Happily, he turned out to be right and lived for seventeen years after the publication of his essay.

Sontag and Gould, both public intellectuals, pushed aside emotional responses to their cancer, opting instead for rigorous arguments derived from their respective fields of study. Actually, Sontag's antipathy to metaphor would have presented an obstacle to any personal narrative. Even in her analytic book, she cannot do without the metaphors she seeks to banish. *Illness as Metaphor* famously opens with the assertion that "Everyone who is born holds dual citizenship, in the kingdom of the well and in the kingdom of the sick." The idea of sickness as a kingdom, the notion that we have two passports: these sorts of figurative formulations repeatedly nudge their way into her prose.

Despite her major role in reducing the stigma surrounding cancer, Sontag's belief that we should and can eliminate all metaphors from our discussion of illness remains quixotic at best. We can no more purge ourselves of metaphors than we can purge ourselves of words. In the years following Sontag's *Illness as Metaphor*, many patients and some caretakers resemble Stephen Jay Gould in contesting their physicians' words by formulating narratives and metaphors about their own case histories.

An overwhelming majority of these publications are memoirs, the focus of this wide-ranging chapter on an astounding proliferation of books. The message of each of these zillions of memoirs is the variation: the singularity of every unique case. Yet when read together, they show the individuals posited by the genre striking out on similar paths. So hang on to your hat: to chart these routes I'll have to romp through them. But first, I pick a work about prostate cancer as a model to delineate the cancer memoir's traditional structure. Then, mapping the roads taken by many memoirists, I consider what we gain by reading the accounts of patients furiously denouncing the medical establishment or fearfully envisioning the nature of an appalling disease. In the rest of this chapter, I turn to reinventions of the memoir in humorous and graphic books as well as hybrid forms that are hardly recognizable as memoirs.

Far from being the cause of cancer, roiling anger—or its twin, churning fear—may be the effect of diagnosis and treatments. Beyond providing us company in misery, what are the rewards of reading this often angry or fearful work? As readers, we derive pleasure from observing vulnerable individuals like ourselves who are talking back to the experts, releasing pent-up emotions, gaining some sort of control over situations of vertiginous vulnerability, and instructing us on ingenious ways to name or picture perilous circumstances. Forming a considerable corpus, patient and caregiver memoirs offer an incisive exploration and critique of contemporary cancer culture.

Let's take Michael Korda's *Man to Man* to lay bare the pattern that can be found in memoirs about every form of cancer. Cancer memoirs tend to move from the discovery of suspicious symptoms and detection to diagnosis, from finding and initiating a series of treatment to enduring them, from distress over body dysfunction or disfigurement to recuperation and recovery or recurrence and the approach of death. With some variations, Korda, then the editor in chief of a major publishing house, shaped this plot to contend that men know much less about prostate cancer than women do about breast cancer. In *Man to Man*, he attempts to persuade other men to arm themselves with knowledge. To use the language of Vivien Gornick—a specialist in the genre who makes a distinction between the "situation" of a memoir and its "story"—the situation or context of *Man to Man* is prostate cancer; the story conveying the writer's emotional investment concerns the much-needed education of men. Here's how Korda works the memoir template.

- *Discovery and detection.* After a biopsy, a voice on the phone speaking the word "unfortunately" informs Michael Korda of his diagnosis and the need to schedule all sorts of scans to see if his prostate cancer has spread. Since he immediately wonders how long the cancer existed before detection, a flashback informs us of the years before his 60th birthday, when an enlarged prostate caused frequent urination and a series of earlier biopsies taught him about the indignities of treatment. Infections from an ultrasound probe that "looked like the end of an old-fashioned bedpost" or a "monstrous dildo," fatigue, and urinary problems conclude the flashback and return us to his cancer diagnosis, but now with the worrisome assumption that if he had gone to Memorial Sloan-Kettering eighteen months earlier, his tumor would have been found at a more treatable stage. Converted to the importance of PSA testing (which some medical authorities question), he believes that men should be as vigilant about getting their PSA taken on a regular basis as women have become about annual mammograms.

- *Finding and initiating treatment.* While conversations with survivors, consultations with specialists, and second opinions bombard him with conflicting advice, the suspense of *Man to Man* hinges on a frightful question: will Michael Korda's decision to opt for a radical prostatectomy leave him incontinent, impotent, or both? His resolution to travel from New York to Baltimore so as to gain access to a surgeon expert in a "nerve-sparing" procedure (which offers the possibility of recovered potency) depends on his excellent job and equally excellent health insurance. He underscores the threat to livelihood that prostate cancer poses to less fortunate men and also the difficulty that most men experience in speaking about incontinence and impotence. His book seeks to talk bluntly, "man to man," about the ways "prostate cancer will try your soul and the soul of the partner who loves you." Korda rises to the challenge by revealing that while making love to his wife the night before surgery, he realized that "it would never *feel* like this again": "the familiar excitement of ejaculation, the spurt of semen, the deep peace that comes with orgasm and the feel of one's own body liquids." Since "the reality of sex is fluid, liquid, wet," what sort of sex would sex be without the discharge of semen and seminal fluids?

- *Enduring treatment.* Although the surgery is successful, a malfunctioning pain-controlling machine in the Johns Hopkins Hospital left

Korda exhausted and desperate for relief. And a leaking Foley catheter made him feel "shamed, humiliated, soiled, no longer an adult in full control of my bodily functions." Relieved but also terrified by release from the hospital and the logistics of travel, he again seems typical when he fearfully realizes that recuperation at home places the burden of management squarely on himself. Despite excellent hired helpers, the catheter gives him a preview of incontinence: "It meant that there wasn't a moment, day or night, that you weren't *conscious* of your urine, weren't thinking about it, weren't concerned that you were leaking it, or dripping it, or that other people could smell it on you, no matter how much you washed, and scrubbed the catheter tube with alcohol pads, and sprayed Lysol everywhere around you." Without a timetable, post-surgical problems lack the drama of diagnosis and surgery.

- *Distress over bodily dysfunction and recuperation.* Like many patients, Korda looks in the mirror and sees someone elderly: "a stranger, an old man from my posture to the dark bags under my eyes." Explosions of rage punctuate mishaps with leakage. When the catheter finally comes out, he relies on a walking regimen, Kegel exercises (to strengthen the muscles around the sphincter), excursions with his wife, and conversations with other survivors until he can remove his Depends diapers and put on Sir Dignity briefs. By the end of his narrative, the necessity of having to wear a pad and an occasional spurt of urine do not seem to warrant further surgery. And during a visit to a sexual function center, an injection that produces a painful erection teaches him the distinction between erection and arousal. He can become more philosophical about the various implants and pump devices that he might or might not want to attempt in the future. Nine months after surgery and declared cancer-free, Korda experiences what he defines as recovery: the dawning realization that "cancer was an *episode* in one's life, neither the end of it nor, more important, the whole of it."

In his reactions to the medical establishment, the nature of cancer, and their combined injuries—the topics that take up the attention of most memoirists and the bulk of this chapter—Michael Korda is also prototypical. Throughout *Man to Man*, he names the influential specialists with whom he confers. He profits from their expertise; however, he finds that these imperious physicians gloss over the physical consequences of treatments, misinform patients, or communicate ineffectively. Korda comes to believe that "surgeons don't necessarily know how it feels to be on the receiving end," as patients do. Although the doctors he consulted "pooh-poohed my questions about home nursing care," he finds it critical. Worse, his surgeon's parting advice against excessive fluid intake lands him in the ER with a blockage that neither suppositories nor enemas can alleviate. Weeks after the prostatectomy, Korda is "thunderstruck" when a local doctor tells him what his Hopkins surgeon had neglected to mention: that he had been able to spare only one of the two nerve-bundles.

Because at the end of his memoir Korda must continue dealing with incontinence and impotence, he deploys the common image of cancer as an implacable aggressor with the sobering conviction that "to defeat cancer you have to destroy a part of yourself." Surgeons refer to the operation site as "the field" and oncologists consider themselves "in the trenches" because "cancer is personalized, with good reason, as the *enemy*: cunning, swift-moving, deadly, giving no quarter, taking no prisoners." Conscious of all the collateral damage, Korda attributes the disappearance of some of his friends to their fear. The silence of friends contrasts with his own obsessive thinking about cancer, which, "like war, is such a big event in anybody's life that it tends to blot out everything else for a long time." During the battle, "there's a certain exhilaration of the kind which invariably accompanies war, a powerful adrenaline rush that sees one through the worst of it." There is victory—"but look at what we sacrificed to win, and was the sacrifice really necessary?"

Throughout *Man to Man*, references to stuffable erections, dry ejaculations, urine leaks, and castration emphasize the damaged body. After surgery, Korda finds himself unprepared for "the ways in which the least interesting and most normal of everyday bodily functions had taken over my life, almost to the exclusion of everything else." Tubes, drains, catheters, bedpans, urinals, leak-proof mattress covers, protective floor mats, diapers, and diaries of urine output eclipse all other concerns. The debilitating consequences of his operation fuel his skepticism about future surgical interventions. Yet experience of the damaged body also unites the men in his support group—"We were all in this together, knights of the Maxipad and the condom catheter"—and intensifies intimacy. About cancer, Korda believes that "the one thing it *does* do is to create a genuine camaraderie." For these men, as for veterans, "survival is a powerful bond."

Keeping the shape of the memoir in mind, we can start to fathom its predominant themes by considering a notable element percolating in many: namely, fury at the medical establishment. Historically, doctors have generally confronted miserable images of themselves in literature. Frustration—like Michael Korda's over his dependency on the physicians he criticizes—fuels the memoirs that multiplied while sophisticated technologies evolved in the field of biomedicine. Quite a few books, authored by privileged professionals lucky to consider cancer "an episode" from which they can extrapolate lessons, contain what the sociologist Arthur Frank calls quest stories: they use illness as "the occasion of a journey" to discover "what can be gained through the experience." As the genre evolved, however, some patients and caregivers departed from the quest plot to dwell on the distress of terminal disease. Others steer between the standard conclusion of either recovery or imminent death, as I did in my memoir.

Whether in recovery, end-of-life, or inconclusive stories, though, memoirists tackle inadequate doctoring, medical mistakes, alienating hospital environments, economic burdens, and imponderable decision-making that baffle patients confined within ever-circumscribed lives. Even when doctors receive praise for their skill and integrity, their training and the conditions under which they must work are thought to compromise compassionate care. Although I was in a roiling rage while composing parts of my own memoir, I was surprised and exhilarated at the intensity of the responses I encountered from patients depleted by a range of treatments and environment quite different from the ones I had experienced.

Excoriating the medical establishment, innumerable memoirists—whether they believe themselves to be cured, curable, or incurable—deem malignant the mortifications to which cancer patients are subjected. When descriptions of dehumanizing ordeals mount, it can be deeply satisfying to read scorching words attesting to energizing and very human outrage.

Since technology robbed the essayist Anatole Broyard of "the intimacy" of his illness, made it "not mine but something that belongs to science," he longed for a doctor who could "repersonalize it" for him. Actually, he wanted more—a doctor with style, magic, skill at interpreting illness with critical acumen, one who understands the panic beneath the mask of patient cheerfulness and who broods over or bonds not with the generic patient but with the individual person. Admittedly, "The sick man asks far too much, he is *im*patient in everything," but especially with the physician who remains encased in "the cadaver of his professional persona."

Broyard's diagnosis of the moribund medical professional comes with a prescription: the doctor can save himself only if he comes "to see that his silence and neutrality are *unnatural*." Should he exchange his authority for his humanity, he would learn to love his work and share with his patient "the wonder, terror, and exaltation of being on the edge of being." While Broyard delighted in envisioning the physician he would have wanted to encounter, other memoirists deplore the doctors to whom they have been consigned or, sometimes worse, the doctors they have chosen.

Barbara Creaturo, youthful and well-connected through her editorial work at *Cosmopolitan* magazine, set out to find cutting-edge researchers to deal with her ovarian cancer, but her wrath at the uncaring care she received caused the editors of her book to fictionalize the names of all the physicians and hospitals. After negotiating a "treacherous landscape mined with misinformation" from several oncologists, Creaturo engaged a "daredevil doctor" who lied in order to get her enlisted in a trial of his drug and then administered doses "far higher" than she deemed proper until she suffered a complete physical breakdown.

Disillusioned, she fulminates against "doctors who'll put your life on the line for a cheap ego thrill, for the pleasure they'll get from stepping onto a podium one day and saying I, *I* discovered the cure for this disease." Toward the end of her memoir, Creaturo asks herself what conclusions she draws from her experience: "That the ethics of cancer researchers are badly frayed? Yes. That life-saving therapies are buried by bureaucratic inefficiency and lost to internecine rivalries among physicians? Again, yes. Patients' needs often come a distant second to the hunger for funding and prestige."

More frequently, anger is triggered by the lapse, caused by misdiagnosis, between detection and discovery. Marianne A. Paget composed a series of essays about the medical mistakes she suffered. The errors of two physicians meant that her sarcoma went undiagnosed until it had metastasized. Paget's earlier sociological study of the blunders inevitably made by physicians forecasted her fate, but it also helped her come to terms with it: "Had I not known about the prevalence of error in medicine, I would not have been able to process what has happened to me without bitterness." More recently, S. Lochlann Jain embedded her account of a late-stage breast cancer—misdiagnosed for three years by three physicians—in an anthropological study of America's cancer culture. According to Jain, "doctors often work under the misguided assumption that cancer is a disease of older people, leading to an immorally high number of delayed diagnoses and, in turn, the large proportion of late-stage cancers."

While Jain dropped her malpractice suit, Paget never pursued one, for she found herself overwhelmed by the disease and by the alienation she felt in observing it on screens in the Dana-Farber radiology department: "I, as an observer, read the signs of my condition from outside. The image projected from inside my body tells me its tale and I, who live in my body, tell mine."

Not mistakes but uncaring care fire up the author Reynolds Price. Although at the close of Price's *A Whole New Life* he emerges free of spinal cancer and convinced that his life has improved, he castigates an unnamed radiation oncologist "who gave the unbroken impression, over five weeks, of being nothing so much as a nuclear physicist whose experimental subjects were, sadly for them, human beings." Price cannot understand why his doctor shied away from involvement. Insufficient training cannot explain the absence of a "frank exchange of decent concern": "When did such a basic transaction between two mammals require postgraduate instruction beyond our mother's breast?"

The "frozen oncologist" instills a "phobia of returning to medical care," even though Price understands "the lamentably drastic limits" of medical training as well as the long hours that drain physicians who deal with anxious people. Yet "surely a doctor should be expected to share—and to offer at all appropriate hours—the skills we expect of a teacher, a fireman, a priest, a cop, the neighborhood milkman or the dog-pound manager," for these are "merely the skills of human sympathy." When Price finally enters rehab—to learn how to survive as a quadriplegic—one of its "liberations" consists of "the general absence of doctors."

That traditionally trained specialists remain either indifferent to pain or ignorant of alternative methods of pain management infuriates a number of memoirists. At a pain clinic, Price discovers nothing but debilitating drugs: "the help of the Pain Clinic stopped there, where so many American physical problems are grounded by doctors who've blindly or willfully impoverished their humane intelligence—on prescription blanks." After pain-obsessed years of "a narcotized life" and another operation, his "spinal cord increased its howling as new scar tissue formed and pressed on already crushed nerves."

Only after a third operation did his surgeon mention the biofeedback training that might have given him earlier relief. Hypnosis and daily writing were methods of dealing with pain that he found on his own. Understandably, Price's final advice for people with cancer contains an explosive metaphor of the person who emerges out of the ordeal: "Grieve for a decent limited time over whatever parts of your old self you know you'll miss" and then "find your way to be somebody else, the next viable you—a stripped-down whole other clear-eyed person, realistic as a sawed-off shotgun and thankful for air."

Also horrified by inadequate pain management, Le Anne Schreiber describes the bewilderment of her mother after an operation on the older woman's pancreatic cancer, as pain reduced her to a drugged and bedridden existence. A celiac block only intensified the need for more painkillers. "Why must medicine feel so much like a hit and run accident?" her daughter wonders in *Midstream.* Only after a friend mentions an oncologist who uses a TENS machine—sending electrical pulses to targeted nerves—does Mrs. Schreiber receive some relief. Ironically, she had first resisted consulting Dr. Ye because she believed that she did not need an oncologist. Her previous physician had told her, "You are cured. You are no longer a cancer patient." No wonder Mrs. Schreiber and her daughter remained baffled by her continual loss of weight and strength.

*Midstream* suggests that too many oncologists remain reluctant to specify a prognosis, or they conceal it. Amid innumerable and indeterminate tests, Mrs. Schreiber begins to blame herself for not recuperating. Part of the problem is patient denial; however, even her daughter seems mystified as Mrs. Schreiber loses all vestiges of autonomy. Only when she has clearly begun to die do they learn that metastases had spread throughout the stomach, liver, and chest cavity. Le Anne Schreiber's brother, a doctor, knew that "the surgeon had seen fluid leaking from the pancreatic tumor into Mom's abdominal cavity during the operation and he included that information in his report," but the brother—like the physician who pronounced Mrs. Schreiber "cured"— had "chosen not to undermine our hope with his knowledge." A similar combination of patient denial and physicians' insistence on withholding a prognosis tortures the historian Gerda Lerner in her account of her husband's malignant brain tumor.

In the ironically titled *A Very Easy Death*, Simone de Beauvoir provided the prototype of a miserable death caused in part by the doctors' determination to conceal cancer from the patient. Seeing her mother's misery, Beauvoir wanted to rescue her from the tormenting physicians: "Get a revolver somehow: kill Maman: strangle her." Similarly outraged, Stan Mack—in a prose account with drawings, titled *Janet & Me*—depicts the burdens of managing critical care for a partner who refused "to live in cancerland at all." In one of his drawings, a blank large box—with the hint of a tail or an eye in the lower right-hand corner—represents "the proverbial invisible elephant living in our apartment"; subsequent drawings delineate bedpans, commodes, wheelchairs, ambulances, and hospital beds.

Here, as elsewhere, the denial of the patient is buttressed by the denial of the doctor, who refuses to answer any messages or see the patient after the case has become terminal. Like Stan Mack, readers are left feeling that "doctors avoided giving us information that would have made what was left of Janet's life easier for all of us." At least their doctor referred Janet to hospice, an advisor acknowledges: "Some keep doing chemo as the body is being taken to the undertakers."

The memoirs composed by doctor-patients prove that the chasm between those who treat and those who need treatment impairs all concerned. After innumerable delays, misread films, misdiagnoses, and botched procedures, the anesthesiologist Allen Widome—who had been told that he was "a hypochondriac complaining about a non-existent ailment"—finally discovered that he was suffering from lymphoma that had metastasized from the spleen to the bowel, the diaphragm, and the kidney. Dr. Widome's memoir fulminates against the uncaring attitudes of hospital personnel, the long wait periods, the unnecessary repetition of often inconclusive tests, the conflicting advice of experts, and especially the fact that physicians fail to give the words of their patients sufficient weight.

Dr. Edward Rosenbaum's *A Taste of My Own Medicine*, more sophisticated than its movie adaptation *The Doctor*, rails against multiple misdiagnoses that delayed the treatment of his larynx cancer for nine months—his symptoms were also attributed to psychological problems—and that would have been grounds for "a good malpractice suit," had he chosen to pursue it. Instead Rosenbaum becomes a patient-advocate in a book that decries inordinately long wait times, skimpy gowns that expose and infantilize adults, unresponsive or inaccessible physicians, old and malfunctioning radiation machinery, and American hospitals' reliance on big-business models. When his X-ray treatments produce a case of shingles, Rosenbaum sees himself as "a victim of iatrogenic disease, a disease caused by medical treatment."

Concerned about mistreatment and its expenses, Rosenbaum points out that the itemized charges on hospital bills cannot be comprehended even by doctors and that Medicare's billing processes remain not only incoherent but inconsistent. Profits have replaced patients as the major concern of medical institutions dedicated to marketing, public relations, and the "dumping" of uninsured people. From start to finish, Rosenbaum believes, "the physician and the patient are not on the same track."

Much more moderate in tone, Dr. Fitzhugh Mullan's *Vital Signs* nevertheless presents horrific justification for a malpractice suit he did not pursue. A biopsy of a mass in his chest had bled, "necessitating an emergency thoracotomy—a chest-splitting procedure that opens the thorax down the front and around under the breast to the back." Questioning what caused the bleeding and the difficult operation "would have seemed like an affront—an ungrateful challenge to the same people who were keeping me alive." But the surgery severed his right phrenic nerve, rendering his right lung function-less, and eventually resulted in an infection-filled cavity in his sternum that required a succession of perilous reoperations. During this passage through a "medical gulag," Mullan considered himself an iatrogenic catastrophe. He never received a complete account of the initial event or its complications, which "could have cleared up some of the divided feelings I had about the care I received."

When newspaper articles reported Mullan's disenchantment with the depersonalized care he received, he was "stunned at the gap" between physicians angry at his exposé and patients heartened by his comments on "the paucity of human touch and understanding amidst the modern therapies for cancer and other illnesses." Minding the gap, another doctor-patient, Janet R. Gilsdorf, attributes that paucity of touch and understanding to "Wal-Mart medicine":

> I'm furious at the current mess in the medical system; upset that, for lack of money, patients can't get the basic care they need; angry that physicians have been herded with economic whips into systems that seem to serve administrators and third-party payers rather than ill people; frustrated with the layers of bureaucracy that separate doctors from their patients.

The magazine editor Katherine Russell Rich—after a misdiagnosis taught her that she had to "behave like a consumer" to get good care—became wary of "lawsuit medicine." Her oncologist had refrained from explaining that metastases had cracked one of her ribs; then this doctor became worried about a lawsuit and refused to continue treating Rich, effectively firing her.

Skyrocketing financial burdens inflicted by the "mess in the medical system" take center stage in the journalist Amanda Bennett's

*The Cost of Hope.* Years after her husband's death, she still did not know exactly what specific form of kidney cancer killed him, even though they had consulted six pathologists, four hospitals, and three oncologists. After seven years of treatment, however, she finally does realize that his treatment came to more than $600,000. The delay in her comprehension of the cost arose from "voluminous and often incomprehensible" bills, huge disparities between the amounts paid by insurance companies and the amounts billed by hospitals, and radically variant percentages of money added on by different hospitals and doctors for drugs. "What can we do about a system in which neither the people who pay—our employers—nor the people who use the services—Terence and I and everyone like us—can really see or influence the cost?" Bennett's book helps explain why cancer patients are twice as likely as other Americans to go bankrupt.

The most searing indictment of the "mess in the medical system" of a specific cancer hospital appears in the actor Evan Handler's account of his recovery from leukemia in *Time on Fire.* Handler, who underwent several cycles of chemotherapy, denounces the sloppy and heartless treatment he received at Memorial Sloan-Kettering, a world-class research institution where "there were not enough pillows and blankets to go around. Sheets and pillowcases were stained and in shreds." The catastrophic shortage of nurses and physicians resulted in dismissive, distracted, and sometimes dangerous doctoring. His rage against the inflated egos and insensitivity of the medical staff erupts periodically.

When Handler subsequently receives a bone marrow transplant at Johns Hopkins, also a research institution, he marvels at landing "on another planet," where everyone makes an effort "to treat each patient as an invaluable resource." But an infection lands him back in Sloan-Kettering, and a succession of crises—the building's plumbing problem, a three-day delay in removing an infected catheter, mistakes in the fever charts, a doctor who callously convinces him that his life is effectively over—testify to "the savage indifference" he decries.

Handler's terrors explain why at one point he "started dreaming, every night, about executing the entire staff of Sloan-Kettering with a machine gun." Temperamentally incapable of relinquishing control over his body, Handler expresses impatience markedly different from the whimsical perspective of the psychologist Dan Shapiro, who describes his bone marrow transplant at a different hospital under more auspicious circumstances. Yet when a team of physicians whom Shapiro had not met appears in his room to discuss his case as if he were some sort of ethnographic artifact, when he cannot get their attention or even their names, he reaches for his "trusty friend"—"the ultimate in water weaponry: fake chrome barrel, black trigger, orange tubes wrapped around the handle"—and is delighted to interrupt the resident who says "So, in summary, this is a twenty-three-year-old Caucasian male with—AN UZI!"

Eve Ensler shares Evan Handler's fury at Memorial Sloan-Kettering, where she arrived having to deal with an intra-abdominal abscess, an ileostomy (requiring a pouch to collect excrement), and daunting decisions to be made about further treatment for uterine cancer. This last problem of decision making haunts many memoirists, who ask, "Isn't suffering from cancer enough? Why must I simultaneously make the most difficult decisions of my life?" The playwright's memoir, *In the Body of the World*, describes the repeated insertion of drainage tubes that feel like garden hoses while doctors ask her to consider radiation. Why, she thinks, "are you even thinking of radiation if it could destroy my intestines and make it impossible for me to eat or poop again?"

Her doctor's response—"It's up to you"—baffles her. So Ensler asks what he would do in her situation and "he says, 'Can't say.'"

His cavalier attitude—convincing her that she has dwindled into an irrelevance—ignites her ire "at the institutions that are meant to heal and support the sick and suffering but don't even see them," at "the blaming radiologist, the rock-and-roll catheter surgeon, the sadist-late-for-dinner doctor dude, the bruises all over my arms from over-worked and underpaid, bitter nurses." She puts one hand on her ileostomy bag and the other on her drainage bag: "My bags are holsters. Inside are guns instead of pus and shit, and I pull them fast and aim-bang-fire Sloan-Kettering."

A book Evan Handler published a few years after his memoir shows that he eventually learned to moderate his anger. Glimpsing, upon his return to Sloan-Kettering, the doctor he had "represented as the most malevolent creature in the story of my survival," he sees that the man looks nothing like what he remembered. Wondering if he might have twisted other events, Handler realizes that his earlier rage—though not unfounded—may have been misdirected, for "the indignity of illness is the severest one I've ever known."

At some point, many survivors and caretakers come to the conclusion of Adam Wishart, whose history of cancer science forms a counterpoint to his account of his father's dying with metastases from a primary site that the doctors fail to find: "The failure of medicine was not the fault of the doctors." But given the mistakes, obfuscations, mortifications, uncertainties, and suffering of treatment, how can one not round up the usual suspects? How can one not feel as if—in the immortal words of Emily Dickinson—one's life has stood a loaded gun?

Maybe because we intuit that none of these memoirists would be likely to fund-raise for the NRA, reading about such righteous indignation can be oddly thrilling, for its invigorating dynamism offsets the grotesque abjection and submission inflicted on patients. And along with the memoirists as well as their physicians, we can hope that some of the problems they encountered and targeted have been solved and that others will be. As a famous rabbi once impatiently asked, admittedly in a totally different context, "If I am not for myself, who will be for me? But if I am for myself only, what am I? And if not now, when?"

The flip side of anger at treatment is fear of cancer. Those memoirists who turn their attention from identifiable professionals (trying to help) toward inchoate forces (setting out to harm) must decide whether to enlist in a dangerous struggle against an unknown. Reading their panicky accounts produces a different sort of reward, one related to the profound gratification of finding words that express what cannot be fathomed, for patients have created a complex vocabulary to describe the mysterious presence of cancer and their relationships to it.

While I was writing my memoir, my sense of being invaded—but by what exactly?—led me to search in my reading for the analogies that helped other people conceptualize what was besieging the self: not a stalwart "I" but a compromised "me." Gruesome as the memoirists' metaphors of cancer are, they clarify the puzzling nature of this disease and how it feels to contend with it. So much for Susan Sontag's strictures!

Because cancer often remains unseen and unfelt for months before its detection, patients find it necessary to visualize the insidious but furtive development of unregulated cells. Something, a not-me, lurks within me, seeking my annihilation, even at the expense of its own existence. For this reason, many memoirists think of cancer as the sneaky alien within: an it-in-me. Peppered throughout innumerable books, references to a virtual bestiary cast the mysterious presence of cancer as a cockroach, a termite, a worm, or a crab. Like a corroding house, the body has been infested. When cancer grows, it feels like a gnawing rat, a fanged snake, an eel, a raging bull, a wild horse, an insatiable beast, a voracious panther, biding its time, or an octopus with far-flung tentacles. If not an uncontrollable animal, cancer is a wilding thug, a stalking gunman, a bunch of juvenile delinquents, a munching gargoyle, or an insatiable parasite.

The interloper feeds off healthy organs to strengthen itself. About his cancer, a dying Gordon Stuart mourned, "There is something not me in me, an 'it,' eating its way through the body." On learning of her disease, the poet Alicia Ostriker exclaimed, "I don't want to be eaten alive." By focusing on the imperialism of the not-me-in-me, Dr. Siddhartha Mukherjee explains the dread accompanying the image of cancer as a foreign cannibal: "Cancer is an expansionist disease; it invades through tissues, sets up colonies in hostile landscapes, seeking 'sanctuary' in one organ and then immigrating to another." The idea of unbridled and unpredictable spreading horrifies patients with the prospect of a painfully protracted demise from a disease that originates in one organ but can migrate anywhere.

When the body has been occupied by an invading colonizer, even peace-loving patients may enlist in a fight to save their lives. After surgeries for breast cancer as well as a glioblastoma, the fashion model and photographer Lynn Kohlman produced *Lynn Front to Back*, a photo-narrative that features pictures of herself as an androgynous and vulnerable but determined warrior. Wearing only briefs in one, she displays her scarred flat chest, protruding ribs, bandaged wrists, and a gaunt face topped by a Mohawk necessitated by the thirty-seven titanium staples evident in her scalp. These are "the marks and the scars of battles" as well as "the rewards of what I conquered": "I had been slammed to the ground and thrown down an abyss. Now I envisioned picking myself up and emerging a samurai warrior, sword in hand." Her treatment fatigue, like battle fatigue, takes on poignancy in light of her wounded, pierced, and gaunt body.

While righteously enlisted in a good war, some memoirists feel bombarded not only by murderous cancer but also by counterattacking medical forces. The traumatized patient enters a terrifying no man's land. A bone marrow transplant shell-shocked the Jungian analyst Christina Middlebrook, who views herself as a "veteran of injury and war and hell." In *Seeing the Crab*, she describes the draconian measures used to attack "the virulence of premenopausal breast cancer": "The technology that has saved me has killed me in order to rescue me." She therefore remembers villages destroyed in Vietnam "in order to save them."

The boy-soldier Middlebrook feels herself to be must take it on faith that the battle has a higher good, even though he contends with friendly fire that is "as apt to kill us as the enemy." His task, like hers: to inch forward, living minute by minute. "By the time the ramp is down and the $35,000 up-front hospital down-payment made, the soldier in me is no longer feisty. Just passive, resigned, beyond thought. I've lost my rifle somewhere and cannot find it."

Although scared, the boy-soldier represents a step up in the evolutionary scale from the zoo creature to which Middlebrook was reduced during the transplant. With a back covered by a pus-filled rash, a sagging left eyelid, and no hair, "the zoo creature does not know if it is a mammal anymore." Unable to swallow, vomiting buckets of blood, "the zoo creature cannot think or remember," cannot watch a video, cannot do anything except hope for a compassionate companion to witness its suffering. If such a witness was absent, Middlebrook needed to disentangle her psyche from her body: "if my body had to die, *I* was not going to accompany it." Middlebrook's sense of self split off from her body. Doused in doses of chemicals, platelets, blood transfusions, diuretics, antinausea and sleeping and pain medications, she found herself "called back" from nullity only by the witnesses "who bore the truth when we could not": "Without the periodic witness . . . who knew who I was," she explains, "*I* could not know myself. Not to know oneself is to die."

The British journalist John Diamond found compassionate witnesses in his family as well as the readers of his London *Times* columns. But when he undertook a succession of grueling surgeries and radiation sessions for throat and oral cancers, he resisted warfare language in part because he knew that the specialists were leading a charge that imperiled his life. Although he rigorously defended standard medical approaches, in his memoir *C: Because Cowards Get Cancer Too . . .* Diamond admitted that his impairments had nothing to do with the disease but were instead "the product of the cure for cancer": a missing lump of tongue, a hole in his throat from a tracheotomy, shooting pains in the neck and jaw, missing saliva glands, loss of voice and taste buds, a limp, edema, overproduction of mucus and saliva, ulcers, a frozen shoulder, toothache, constipation, diarrhea, and radical weight loss.

As the title of his memoir suggests, Diamond did not consider himself courageous; he had not put his own safety at risk for others. Also, "the whole battlefield vocabulary" promulgates the absurd assumption that "brave and good people defeat cancer and that cowardly and undeserving people allow it to kill them."

Of course, popular self-help authors deploy triumphant martial rhetoric in such books as *Knockout, Beating Cancer with Nutrition, A Cancer Battle Plan, How to Fight Cancer and Win, Defeat Cancer Now*, and *Fighting Cancer with Knowledge and Hope*. What subverts this warlike language, however, is the fact that my cancer has been produced by and become part of me; it is not an alien, animal, or cannibal. Somehow and sometimes without any known external trigger, deregulated cell division started in my own healthy cells. For this reason, a number of patients reject combat rhetoric entirely and in the process teach us a lesson about acknowledging disease. Especially while dealing with a chronic or terminal condition, some people decide to reject a bellicose stance that damages the life left to be lived.

During the twenty-nine months between her diagnosis of advanced lung cancer and her death, Deborah Cumming wrote a series of essays on what she called limbo time. A trial drug unexpectedly granted her a reprieve, but she remained acutely conscious of the unknowingness of radiologists, oncologists, and her own self about a cancer they could barely see on their scans and she could rarely feel. Not a coward, deserter, or quitter, Cumming becomes a conscientious objector in *Recovering from Mortality*, for she attempts to make her separate peace—if not with cancer, then with her living and dying. Whereas physicians often urge patients to continue treatment by warning them to "consider the alternative," she determines to dedicate her remaining days or months to more than a war against cancer.

Viewing cancer as "an insistent opportunity to learn that in dying we are alive, in living we are dying," Cumming wanted to consider the alternative. A "good attitude" is not about "fighting, conquering, winning. It's about the daily thankfulness. And about peace, not war." After successful treatment of testicular cancer, Arthur Frank concurred: "Thinking of tumors as enemies and the body as a battlefield is not a gentle attitude toward oneself, and ill persons have only enough energy for gentleness." Because war language can make people dying with cancer feel like losers, it is jettisoned for a pacific response in the accounts of caregivers and patients who, turning to palliative care, opt for comfort when cure becomes impossible. Yet when "the fighting is over," one blogger with incurable cancer feels that she has become "a prisoner-of-war of the side that lost." And when Cumming dreamed, she found herself "in danger from enemies who have guns and intend to shoot and kill me, although there has been no provocation that I know of."

At times, antiwar protestors engage in peaceful resistance, rejecting standard medical care and instead pursuing alternative methods. In an essay called "The Gift of Disease," the postmodernist writer Kathy Acker notes that she feared surgery less than chemotherapy, which at that time began at $20,000. Lacking medical insurance, she refused further treatment after a double mastectomy: "if I remained in the hands of conventional medicine, I would soon be dead, rather than diseased, meat." The passivity and objectification imposed by Western technology horrified her. That traditionally trained doctors demoted her to a puppet meant her death, and therefore her life, would be meaningless. In order not to be reduced to materiality, she turned to psychics, Reichian therapists, Chinese herbalists, and Native American healers, who helped her confront past traumas and unlock the energy that she hoped would heal her. With the excitement and joy they brought her before she died in an alternative Tijuana clinic, cancer became the blocked-me-in-me that needed to be unblocked.

Whether doves or hawks, writers who acknowledge they are dying may view cancer as a not-me-that-has-become-me. Consider that the size of most tumors is often described as if they had been ingested—a pea, a nut, an olive, a lemon, a grapefruit. What is internalized and gestating within the body cannot be digested, but neither can it be expelled. In the British columnist Ruth Picardie's final (unfinished) newspaper article, she recounted the ravages of metastatic breast cancer: "I have become convinced that I am, in fact, pregnant," she confessed: "I need only to refer you to one of the pregnancy manuals dusting up my shelves: the vomiting, the weird stuff growing inside you, the endless waiting for the big day." Another British columnist dying from breast cancer, Dina Rabinovitch, described a night "in death's anteroom" that recalled "that moment toward the end of labour, but still with hours to go, when you utterly reject any lingering notion of natural childbirth and you are yelling for the epidural." To Picardie and Rabinovitch, dying with cancer resembles a labor not unlike birthing, a departure that recalls an arrival. Doulas for the dying are called hospice workers, a reader of my blog once reminded me.

Women with gynecological cancer tend to associate growths in the abdomen with a not-me-that-is-mine: a cancer baby. Eve Ensler tries "to imagine my uterus accommodating this tumor the way it might have once held a baby. I almost had two of them. Babies. Is there a point to a uterus if you do not make a baby? Was the tumor a way of growing something? Was I growing a trauma baby?" Similarly, when Joyce Wadler gets a pelvic sonogram, she hears a "*Whoosh*" from the console: "I know from women's movies on television that this is normally a big moment in sonography, the moment a woman hears her child's heartbeat for the first time, the heralding of a new life. It occurs to me now I may be hearing the opposite. What I am nurturing and carrying inside me may be my own death, or the beginnings of a death: a little death fetus."

The scientific basis for the cancer fetus is explained by the science writer George Johnson in a book that splices an account of his wife's metastatic endometrial cancer with an analysis of multidisciplinary approaches to the disease. Cancer cells "bear a resemblance to those in an embryo—rapidly dividing, chameleon-like, and capable of doing almost anything." Indeed, "an embryo is so much like a tumor that the early days of pregnancy resemble the incursion of a malignant growth." Cancers that borrow "some of the mechanisms of embryogenesis" bring to my mind *Rosemary's Baby,* but to Johnson they resemble the pods taking over the earth in *Invasion of the Body Snatchers.* After seeing that film, the memoirist Dorothea Lynch judged it "a bad choice of movies" for patients: "people losing control of their own bodies, alien plants reproducing cell by cell into duplicate human beings, clinging green tendrils: and everywhere change, change, change."

All the connotations clustered around cancer make anxiety the predominant mood of the memoir. To the journalist Juliet Wittman, fear manifests itself physically when she first feels the lump in her breast, at the biopsy, while waiting for information about lymph node involvement, while deciding which of a complicated menu of protocols she should choose, while dealing with nausea and hair loss from chemotherapy, with fatigue from radiation, with "the choking sensation that threatens to cut off your breath" or "weakness in the knees" or the "feeling that you're lost somewhere in space, turning and turning in the black ether, while slowly, very slowly and starting from the heart, your entire body turns to ice."

Panic accompanies Wittman to the wig store, the Chinese herbalist, the massage therapist, the fortune-teller. Paranoid about any minor bump, she feels guilty for suffering more anxiety after treatment has successfully concluded. Indeed, "fear of recurrence is so intimate" that it resembles "one of those stooped, shambling Dickens characters. You can imagine this creature walking beside you, tugging with clammy hands on your sleeve, blowing decay-scented breath in your face, talking incessantly in a kind of smug, mumbling hiss—a self-chosen familiar who refuses to leave your side."

One locus of fear involves the passive role assigned to patients.

"The very word 'patient' (Latin root, *patior*, 'to suffer') is a give-away," the columnist Max Lerner explains. "Patients suffer things to be done to them, becoming thereby the *acted upon*, the diminished." Although he claims to have rejected this passive assignment throughout treatments for lymphoma and prostate cancer, during much of Lerner's early illness he "felt split between two selves, one, the 'sick' self I had to live *with*, the other the 'normal' one I was trying to live *by*." Indeed, he believes that "a war was being waged between them until the healing could set in and the sick self could become the jumping-off point toward a new balance." In the experience of the less-sanguine Barbara Ehrenreich, the endless exams, scans, and high-tech tests "blurred the line between selfhood and thing-hood," between "organic and inorganic, me and it." For Lerner and Ehrenreich, naming this condition reanimates the stolen "me" that had threatened to degenerate into an "it."

Both before the signs of treatment make the cancer patient visible and after, when those signs disappear or can be hidden, another anxiety clusters around issues of self-disclosure. In *The Summer of Her Baldness*, the visual artist and theorist Catherine Lord likens telling friends about her cancer to "coming out of the closet": "You don't do it just once, and once you've done it you can never stop. It's an act to be repeated again and again in different contexts. Cancer is a disease I can't just have, or be—that would be far too humane—but an identity I must state, or choose not to state, at every encounter." In a series of diary entries and reprinted emails to and from intimates, Lord exploits a persona she calls "Her Baldness" to express the self-dramatizing, operatic person she became after diagnosis. The split between sick HB and healthy Lord signals a pervasive sense of self-division inaugurated by a disease that used to be as unspeakable as homosexuality was several decades ago.

The disease of cancer can still be accompanied by a sense of shame and by economic as well as physical and emotional liabilities. According to Lord, "The cancer closet is at least as complicated as the sexuality closet. You can never get entirely out and you can never get entirely back in." Though her analogy may provoke dissent—a patient coming out of the cancer closet will not be subjected to bullying or denied a religious funeral—it also startles us into new realizations about what the invisibility of cancer signifies.

How can writers possibly make this alarmed story of paranoia and schizophrenia engaging or, harder still, amusing to readers? As the world of the memoirist constricts, it infantilizes patients who are often wary and weary, dependent on specialists with incomprehensible knowledge, reliant on partners or children or parents for physical aid and psychological comfort, unable to nurture their families because they are in need of nurturance themselves. Celebrity memoirists such as Betty Rollins, Lance Armstrong, Jill Ireland, Barbara Barrie, Fran Drescher, and Robin Roberts pique interest by recounting the glamorous events in which they participated, the legendary people in their lives, and their exotic travels and pets and hobbies, often accompanied by glossy photographic inserts. In this case, the pleasure of readers resembles the enjoyment many of us get from *People* magazine.

Throughout *It's Always Something*, Gilda Radner wants to make cancer—"the most unfunny thing in the world"—funny. The book's poignancy hinges on her inability to become the comedienne that cancer needs "to come in there and lighten it up." After the insertion of a tube with a rubber bag of mercury through her nose and down into Radner's digestive tract, she tries to joke about her frustration at excreting it and cleaning up the tiny spheres: "It was quintessential Roseanne Roseannadanna. A wise nurse at the hospital told me later, 'Never let a gynecologist put anything in your nose.'" Yet she ends up feeling "abandoned in nuclear fallout," longing for her lost self; and so she starts to introduce herself with the phrase, "I used to be Gilda Radner." That she had tried every supplementary approach from visualization to crystals and modeled on the cover of *Life* magazine as "a symbol of conquering cancer" only heightened the despair that makes her book so affecting. The effort to be funny in the context of cancer seems audacious and at the same time wrenchingly doomed to failure. Gilda Radner takes on the poignant role of a sad clown, a Pagliacci or Chaplin.

According to the comedian Robert Schimmel's memoir, *Cancer on Five Dollars a Day*, he found it easier to use humor to get through treatment. "Just my luck," Schimmel wisecracked when told he had non-Hodgkin's lymphoma. "I get the one not named after the guy." The joke brings him hope that he can continue doing what makes him feel alive, getting a laugh. He ridicules the "dick wig sales rep" in his hospital room and "Al Qaeda living in my asshole." To evade a speeding ticket, he uses his evident hair and weight loss as "the ultimate *Get Out of Jail Free* card." He kids about "a series of alternative, sometimes far-out *distractions*" like Reiki and crystal therapy.

In stand-up performances, Tig Notaro and Jenny Allen make comedy seem courageous not simply because they are gagging about gagging on stage but also because they must deal (live) with the discomfort of the audience at their broaching the subject of cancer through comedy. Cancer and comedy are not generally supposed to go together.

One of the funnier cancer memoirs is composed by the novelist Joni Rodgers, whose *Bald in the Land of Big Hair* deals with her treatment for non-Hodgkin's lymphoma. Although she is troubled by a series of misdiagnoses and by skyrocketing bills that eventually caused her to declare bankruptcy, Rogers jokes about being "enrolled in a Christian Scientist HMO; apparently, any form of medical intervention was against their religion." Since the oncologist's terms blunt harsh realities, she riffs on the word "alopecia," the clinical word for hair loss: "*The alopecia are in bloom a-gain. Such a delicate flow-ah*" or "Alopecia, gentille alopecia . . . Alopecia, je te plumeria!" A succession of headgears turn her into a series of outré creatures: a delicate silk into a fortune-teller ("Gaze into my crystal ball"), a chiffon into "a pre-*Sunset Boulevard* Carol-Burnett-as-Gloria-Swanson" ("Max, I'm ready for my close-up"), a green beret into "a gay GI Joe," a blue baseball cap into Forrest Gump, and a headwrap into a Ubangi ("Bwana. I bwana have my hair back").

The wisecracking stops when Rodgers considers the collateral damage inflicted on children of cancer patients. In a chapter called "The Queen Has Cancer," Rodgers interweaves her vulnerable son's fairy tale—about rescuing the sick Queen by slaying a dragon and finding the curative magic moss—with episodes of parental incapacity, such as when he had to find a way to unlock the house as she sat in the car too nauseated to move. What emerges is the grief and anger of children at depleted parents who cannot parent and who monopolize all the care and attention as they become physically unrecognizable. Sidestepping self-pity, Rodgers also confronts the social perplexities of patients who become platitude magnets. Targeting pious clichés—"The Lord never gives us more than we can bear" and "If you ask the Heavenly Father for bread, He will not give you a stone"—does not prevent her from connecting to "an undeniably real force that flows from beyond our understanding," but it does protect her from the "deluge of chicken soup for the soul" force-fed to many patients.

Instead of a chronological account, Rodgers produced a series of essays on specific topics to which she brings a range of stylistic techniques. Because she felt disconnected from the diagnosis, for example, she presents it as a *Brady Bunch* TV sit-com, opening with her husband saying "Is that a casaba melon in your neck or are you just happy to see me (Audience laughter.)" In a chapter titled "Passion Slave: Secret Life of a Lymphomaniac," Rogers recounts her lovemaking with her husband (and the chemo pump attached to her body); she decides that she can "still give him something" and so uncouples to engage in oral sex, but immediately gags in recoil. Although she always thought that her sensual essence tasted of plum wine, "It grieved me greatly that my love canal was now more like Love Canal." While returning to a drafted novel during chemotherapy, she finds revision therapeutic, for her fictional characters "became the happy recipients of all the sex I wasn't getting in the real world, every intimate encounter cooked to perfection in the convection oven of my frustration."

In *My One-night Stand with Cancer*, Tania Katan also ridicules her sexual plight. At age 21 at the time of her first mastectomy and then at 30 at the time of her second, she had entered into dysfunctional relationships with the neurotic women who first discover the lumps in her breasts and from whom she must extricate herself. While cutting back and forth between these two periods in her life, Katan jokes about the breast clinic ("a lesbian mixer"), about joking (about "Breast Wishes!" and keeping "abreast of things"), and about her postsurgery chest, which is "grosser than ugly people French-kissing, dirty fingernails, and stepping in dog shit." In a scene evoking Audre Lorde's *Cancer Journal*, she is incredulous when the social worker comes to talk to her about Bosom Buddies, Y-Me, and Cosmetics for Cancer, convinced that the person "can't be for real" and must be a drag queen.

Tania waits in a medical waiting area that looks "like *Queer Eye for the Sick Guy* showed up and said, 'We're thinking *sick* plus *waiting* equals . . . *brown!*'" Worried about sneezing patients and thinking that meditation might ease her fears, she asks herself, "What would Thich Nhat Hanh do?" Her surgeon's most exciting feature is his eye contact, "which is the surgeon equivalent of congenial." Ruling out all the dietary factors said to cause cancer—sugar, fat, meat, genetically modified foods, preservatives—she thinks, "no wonder I'm hungry! What's left? Air? That's it, I'll become a Breatharian." The title of Katan's memoir comes from her best gay boyfriend, who compares cancer to "a one-night stand that turns into a recurring bad date": "Two months in, a lifetime getting out" and "You never know when he's gonna call or leave you alone for good."

At the happily-ever-after ending of this narrative, Tania meets the love of her life, with whom she runs in a succession of marathons. But she also ends up having to deal with the knowledge that she has inherited a genetic mutation increasing her risk for ovarian cancer. In a synagogue, she hears one Dr. Quiet encouraging people of Eastern European Jewish descent to consider BRCA testing. Joking about the need of American Jews "for reassurance"—"sometimes a shower is just a shower"—Tania listens impatiently to all the other questioners, only to find herself shaking and gasping when her turn comes. Dr. Quiet's response—"BRCA-1 carriers have an eighty-five percent chance of developing breast cancer and a forty-percent chance of developing ovarian cancer"—does little to alleviate her math anxiety: How many of those with ovarian cancer will die, and will she be in the 40 percent?

Although most of the people in the audience assume that Tania is too young to understand cancer, she considers herself "a genetic time bomb that might go off any second." To Dina Rabinovitch, the names of these deleterious genes are "bizarre" because "the abbreviation sounds like *bracha*—Hebrew for blessing."

In the cancer comics that started to proliferate in book form at the start of the twenty-first century, cancer and its treatments are whimsically, poignantly, sassily, or savagely satirized. The overt lack of realism in comic drawings makes the genre congenial to the surrealism of the invisible threat of cancer, the weird technologies and effects of treatment, the disruptive pressures put on families, and the off-the-wall responses of acquaintances. At their best, memoirs in comics present a trenchant analysis of cancer culture in American society: the moneymaking industries that sell patients on the idea that they can cure themselves, willful blindness about ecological factors that contribute to rising cancer rates, economic problems resulting from inequitable insurance systems, and the paradox that cancer cures have been implicated in cancer causes. They also provide readers surprising visual analogues for the situations that many of us encounter.

Throughout the whimsical episodes of *Cancer Made Me a Shallower Person*, Miriam Engelberg's befuddled cartoon surrogate sounds like a female Woody Allen and looks like a curly-haired doodle with eyeglasses. A series of one- or two-page black-and-white cartoon sequences spoof the inanity associated with what is now called "pink-washing": the lucrative and opportunistic promotion of consumer goods and services under the banner of the breast cancer ribbon. The glum cartoon character Miriam only feels further alienated by all the hype—of maintaining a positive attitude, running for the cure, signing up for meditation training sessions, support groups, and cosmetic makeovers. She is especially put off by an insanely cheerful radiation technician with a hand puppet and by euphemistic chemo booklets that feature tropical beach scenes. Miriam rejects the usual boosters and decides instead to make cartooning her spiritual practice.

Other aspects of Miriam's shallow path consist of watching reruns of *Judge Judy*, doing crossword puzzles, and obsessing about celebrity gossip, all undertaken to distract herself from the anxiety induced not only by cancer but also by the responses she encounters from acquaintances. While friends ask implicitly blaming questions about her sugar intake, the character Miriam frets about what she might have done to cause her cancer—did she eat too much cheese?—as Engelberg targets self-help platitudes that intensify her loneliness and guilt.

To cope with the weight gain and libido loss caused by early menopause, Miriam tries new shallow solutions—including a porn movie, but she finds herself fast-forwarding through the sex scenes to get back to the plot. Toward the end of the book, after Miriam suffers with metastases to the brain and bone, Engelberg mocks survivor rhetoric that belies dire mortality statistics. A character is shown triumphantly claiming to be a survivor at diagnosis, after various treatments, and finally right before the time of death is about to be pronounced.

Exceptionally poignant about the pressure cancer puts on families, Brian Fies's *Mom's Cancer*, which he started as "a kind of underground journalism" on the Internet, looks less amateurish, more polished and glossy. A series of black-and-white comics record his and his sisters' responses to their mother's metastatic lung cancer. Some of Fies's drawings render the weirdness of the experience through flagrantly unrealistic images. After a physician finds a bloated lymph node on his mother's chest, the family rejoices that it can be biopsied without a brain or lung operation: "What Luck! Mom's so chock-full of malignancy they can tap her like a Vermont maple and collect buckets of oozing cancer syrup from almost ANYWHERE!" The illustration depicts his mother metamorphosed into a tree with her arms upraised, sprouting leaves, and her trunk tapped by spigots on which buckets hang.

Later, in the midst of treatment and in the middle of a family conversation, the eyes of the mother turn from black to white, a marker of the vacuity produced by all the chemicals. Fies switches to orange and yellow color plates to show how people in emergencies "become MORE of what they already are. Like they get SUPER-POWERS." He and his siblings revert to parodies of their younger selves as they compete in efforts to take care of their mother. To illustrate how aggressive doctors calibrate lethal doses of drugs with medications to strengthen the patient and how challenging this equilibrium becomes for his mother, Fies depicts her balancing on a tightrope with a teetering pole.

In a picture of a single piece of a jigsaw puzzle, Fies wonders why such puzzles appear only in cancer waiting rooms: "I think it's because you're here SO OFTEN, sometimes daily, you can place eight or nine pieces, come back tomorrow, and find the same puzzle waiting, a bit more complete." *Mom's Cancer* concludes with color drawings of his sisters packing up his mom for a move to Southern California, though an afterword explains that the steroids she took to prevent brain inflammation eventually killed her.

Larger and much more colorful than the other cancer comics, Marisa Acocella Marchetto's *Cancer Vixen* addresses the question posed on its first page above a reprinted scan of her breast tumor: "What happens when a shoe-crazy, lipstick-obsessed, wine-swilling, pasta-slurping fashion-fanatic, single-forever, about-to-get-married big-city girl cartoonist (me, Marisa Acocella) with a fabulous life finds . . . A LUMP IN HER BREAST?!?" The sassy tone, suiting its original serialized setting in *Glamour*, allows Marchetto to document her adventurous life BC (before cancer) as a cartoonist and reporter for *Talk* magazine and the *New Yorker*.

But it is also accompanied by some astonishing artwork illuminating the blame game generated by diagnosis. A two-page spread, "The Cancer Guessing Game," provides many squares with answers to the question "Why did I get it?": cigarettes, parabens, antibiotics, antiperspirants, being overweight, nuclear reactors, hormones in chickens, hormone replacement therapy, childlessness, and martinis send the player any number of steps back and forth, but perpetually around the board.

On another page, Marchetto has drawn a picture of herself alone at night in her study. Pondering "all the supposed factors that contributed to any breast cancer diagnosis," she thinks, "WHAT THE HELL ARE WE DOING TO OURSELVES?!" At the bottom of the next full page, Marisa looks up from her drawing desk into a starry night in which crowds of children and adults speak to her from cloud banks. They identify themselves: "We're the women from Long Island. There was a breast cancer hotspot in Huntington"; "In California, where I come from, they found brain cancer clusters"; "15 of us come from South Jersey. They found waste products in our water"; "There was a leukemia cluster in Nevada where I lived, too. Jet fuel was dumped into our drinking water from the nearby naval base . . ." One speaker acknowledges that "IT

WAS *NEVER* PROVEN," but their posthumous voices ask, ". . . AREN'T WE *ENOUGH* EVIDENCE?"

Subsequent drawings embellish the multiple sources of Marissa's distress. While she discusses her lack of insurance with her fiancé and he promises to help financially, she grows smaller and smaller in each frame. After she is told that at 43 she would have to abort a fetus conceived during chemo, four frames portray her unborn babies in a starry sky, waving good-bye, disappearing, or saying, "I'm the only one you have time for now, and the clock's tick, tick, ticking." Later, when Marissa is put on tamoxifen, the last baby in the sky vanishes with a poof of smoke.

At work and on a deadline, Marissa cannot concentrate: in a cartoon revision of a painting by Magritte, the portrait of her face features a boob sticking out where each eye should be. A shot of Neulasta prescribed to increase her white blood cell count, with a price tag of $3,500, is pictured as a cement vat on a truck with a spikey shoot. A large "danger" sign opens the section on radiation undertaken "just to be safe." At the bottom of the platform on which Marissa lies beneath the huge machine, a skull with a chef's hat asks, "How about a side of cancer with that cancer?"

Despite its *Sex in the City* panache, then, *Cancer Vixen* satirizes the dire consequences of inequitable insurance coverage and carcinogenic cancer treatments that produce secondary cancers. No wonder that another, more polemical memoirist—S. L. Wisenberg calls herself "Cancer Bitch" and first decides that she does not want "to be like Cancer Vixen who just thinks about shoes and hair"— ends up getting a port "because Cancer Vixen's drawing hand started getting numb from the chemo needles."

There are very few words, absolutely no colors, and many dark images in the most disturbing cancer comic, David Small's *Stitches*, which stretches the graphic memoir into an autobiographical gothic mystery. The paucity of words underscores the voicelessness of the character David, who at 14 underwent an operation to remove his thyroid and a vocal cord. Even before this event, David grows up in a wordless world of angry noise: his mother crashing around the kitchen, his physician father punching a bag in the basement, his brother slamming on a drum set.

Constantly scolded and threatened by sometimes psychotic relatives, the imaginative boy (whose gift is drawing) falls in love with the Alice depicted by John Tenniel in Lewis Carroll's classic children's tales, probably because she also feels too big or too small in a series of menacing scenes populated by querulous or hostile creatures. Riffing on his own last name, the artist repeatedly shows his small character in the large, labyrinthine hospital corridors where his father worked.

Midway through *Stitches*, Small shifts the perspective to magnify the dimensions of David's vocal cords as they should have looked and then the interior of his throat with only one vocal cord. A single image of an open mouth then appears with the only sound David can make after the operation: "ACK." In another frame, we see David looking in the mirror at a "crusted black track of stitches; my smooth young throat slashed and laced back up like a bloody boot." Later still, he discovers a note on his mother's desk saying that "the boy does not know it was cancer": ten frames show him reading the note and trying to take it in.

Voiceless, David grows up feeling invisible, nonexistent, troubled by recurrent nightmares, jailed for driving without a license, running away from school, and furious at his parents' collusion in silence. The cartoon bubble around his words is hyphenated so we sense what his rasping whisper sounds like when he finally responds to their interminable bullying with the question, "Have you nothing to say to me?"

Only a kindly psychiatrist—depicted as the White Rabbit in *Alice's Adventures in Wonderland*, complete with a watch—saves David from self-destruction by telling him the truth: that his mother does not love him. Twelve dark wordless pages follow, depicting his denial and then grief as tears turn into a series of storm clouds and torrential rain over landscapes that disappear into gulfs of splattered water—recalling the lake of tears in which Alice swims.

The malice that characterizes Alice's world emerges in subsequent revelations that explain to David some of the sources of his parents' cruelty. First he finds his mother in bed with a woman and realizes one secret that has deformed her life. Then he discovers that his mother's mother had to be hospitalized in "the state insane asylum." Finally, his incessantly smoking father admits "I gave you cancer": back "in those days," breathing difficulties, sinus conditions, and asthma were treated with "two-to-four-hundred rads."

Drawings of the teenager David merging with the child David strapped onto his father's radiation apparatus preface an image of him moving through a black hole, into a bohemian life, and finally into the world of art, "which has given me everything I have wanted or needed since." After his mother's death, David has a dream that concludes *Stitches*: he is being ushered by her into "the old central state asylum," as she sweeps a path to clear "the way for me to follow." The final page contains no pictures, but two words: "I didn't."

With dialogue and narrative prose as well as framed sequences of pictures, cancer comics represent a more obviously mixed mode than a number of books I have discussed that combine the memoir with anthropology, science history, and photography. But all these works prove the malleability of a form often thought to be formulaic. It therefore seems fitting to conclude with a brief look at hybrid works that illustrate how the pliant cancer memoir has metamorphosed into projects that defy categorization. Throughout conventional memoirs, we encounter references to ecological, spiritual, and educational concerns. But they take center stage in environmental, theological, and pedagogic meditations that prove to be exceptions to the rule: unusually patient texts produced by teachers who minimalize and embed their personal cancer narratives within larger frameworks.

One such series of experiments derives from Rachel Carson's groundbreaking book on an imperiled environment, *Silent Spring*, especially its allusion to the absence of bird songs in a poisoned world. Terry Tempest Williams structured *Refuge* into a series of chapters about birds—burrowing owls, whimbrels, snowy egrets—threatened by the rising levels of the Great Salt Lake during the period her mother was struggling with ovarian cancer. Sadness over the decline of her mother and of the Bear River Migratory Bird Refuge washes over her as she hikes trails, spots birds, and attends to her mother.

Steeped in a Mormon religion rooted "in a magical worldview" and in Joseph Smith's mysticism, Williams comes to believe that "an individual doesn't get cancer, a family does." After her mother's death, while witnessing the Great Salt Lake receding and the reemergence of the bird refuge, she begins to think that a land gets cancer. Brooding over her mother, grandmothers, and six aunts, all of whom had mastectomies, and recounting a dream to her father of a "flash of light in the night in the desert," she discovers that she had in fact seen a "golden-stemmed cloud, the mushroom," when in the car with her family near Las Vegas.

Williams's research into nuclear fallout from atomic testing in Nevada and Utah during the 1950s makes her realize "the deceit" she had been living under: "Children growing up in the American Southwest, drinking contaminated milk from contaminated cows, even from the contaminated breasts of their mothers, my mother—members, years later, of the Clan of One-Breasted Women." Her elegiac commemoration of her mother and her mother's land raises awareness about cancer's causes in order to engage Americans in cancer prevention. Similarly, Sandra Steingraber's *Living Downstream*—which argues that cancer cells are not born, but made by pollutants—interpolates a number of personal narratives within its scientific inquiry: about a friend's death from a rare cancer of the spinal cord and Rachel Carson's struggle with breast cancer as well as the author's own diagnosis, in her twenties, of a bladder cancer that she believes to have been environmentally caused.

An illness story is also submerged in a remarkable book addressing the spiritual concerns punctuating many traditional memoirs. Christian Wiman brackets *My Bright Abyss*, a series of essays on poetry, theology, and mysticism, with a preface in which he explains that his thoughts evolved under the shadow of a rare and incurable blood cancer and a conclusion documenting a bone marrow transplant that brought him a long remission. Living without a clear prognosis forces Wiman to reevaluate his alienation from his fundamentalist upbringing and to search for new ways to speak about God. Not the words "omnipotence" and "omniscient" but rather the word "contingency" describes his sense of the divine. And yet honesty compels him to admit that the unimaginable pain of successive treatments "seemed to incinerate all my thoughts of God and to leave me sitting there in the ashes, alone." Later, he concedes, the pain of "too much cancer packed into" his bone marrow "islands" him.

A poet, Wiman takes issue with a famous line by Wallace Stevens—"Death is the mother of beauty." The idea that awareness of death concentrates life so we can treasure it lost its power on Wiman's 39th birthday, when he found himself "looking through the *actual* lens of death." The cancer diagnosis did not heighten but attenuated his world. Everything and everyone felt "far away," "muffled." Turning away from abstractions about death, Wiman goes in search of imaginative languages that intensify a singular aspect of reality which acquires "a life in excess of itself," so "what we feel is more complicated than joy."

Poetry becomes "integral to any unified spiritual life": it preserves the continuity as well as the loss of what it invokes, "because to name is to praise and lose in one instant." Even after a miserable hospitalization, "breathless because of my useless blood, tethered twenty-four hours a day to multiple chemotherapies, angered into someone I hardly recognize and do not like," Wiman can turn to a poem by Ted Hughes and find his faith renewed.

Not belief, but faith—"a motion of the soul toward God"—accompanies Wiman's traumatic experiences: "the God that comes at such moments may not be simple at all, arises out of and includes the very abyss that man would flee." Although pain can replace God—when we pray that "it ease up ever so little"—it leads him to define himself as a Christian: because of the crucifixion, not the resurrection. Christ "felt human destitution to its absolute degree; the point is that God is *with us*, not beyond us in suffering": "I'm suggesting that Christ's suffering shatters the iron walls around individual human suffering, that Christ's compassion makes extreme human compassion—to the point of death, even—possible." Wiman's faith stands in marked contrast to the secularism, the secular Judaism, and the New Age spirituality more often avowed by cancer memoirists, even as it underscores their quest for spiritual insights into suffering.

The late publications of the celebrated literary scholar Eve Kosofsky Sedgwick illuminate the quest for a spiritual response to an incurable illness as undertaken by a non-Christian whose life-work entailed exploring and affirming queer sexuality. Sedgwick's *A Dialogue on Love* recounts her progress in psychotherapy from her depression after a mastectomy and chemotherapy to her confrontation with metastases; however, once again cancer is sidelined, in this case so that she and her therapist can discuss how it triggered anxieties dating back to her chubby and precocious childhood self, her fears and fantasies of punishment, her tendency to identify with anyone except herself.

Cancer reveals to Sedgwick, as it did to Alice James, her "wish of not living," her experiencing "so little attachment to life," her desire to be told *"you can stop now."* In a book that mixes poetry with her therapist's notes and Sedgwick's responses to their sessions, she grapples with the family dynamics that fractured her sexuality between missionary intercourse with her husband and lurid fantasies of pain and shame.

Not all these problems get neatly solved, but through Sedgwick's affection for her therapist, her newfound sensual experiences of her own body, and her tactile experiments with textiles and weaving she resolves a number of issues and redefines love, which becomes a matter of realizing that "another person represents our own access" to transmissible truths and heightened modes of perception. Her queerness in her biological family helps explain and affirm the love and acceptance she achieved as a straight woman in a family of gay men. Working to give up (and help her friends give up) hope and fear about her fate, she experiments with a Buddhist meditation to spark tenderness and gratitude: imagining that each of the people in a public space has been, in some earlier life, her mother. When she studies Sogyal Rinpoche's *Tibetan Book of Living and Dying*, Sedgwick finds Buddhism's embrace of nonbeing more congenial than the Western stress on individual survival.

In subsequent essays, Sedgwick believes that "nothing dramatizes the distance between knowledge and realization as efficiently as diagnosis with a fatal disease." Within the "bardo" of dying—the Tibetan term for an in-between state—she appreciates Buddhist pedagogy, for it subsumes "knowing" to "realizing" how "to unbe a self" or how to be "liberated by both possibility and impossibility, and especially by the relative untetheredness to self" since "No one fails to die: at best, one can get out of one's way." She wanted to practice not Elizabeth Bishop's "art of losing" but rather a mystical "art of loosing," which involves "an emptying-out of the sense of self, a general letting go of one's sense of specialness, of possession, or even of individuality."

Throughout her late essays, Sedgwick accepts herself as a learner and rejects the idea of recovery, especially the idea of recovering the self before diagnosis. "If I can fit the pieces of this self back together at all," she declares in *A Dialogue on Love*, "I don't want them to be the way they were." Like many others, she seeks to use cancer as an opportunity "to be realer."

The tradition traced here reveals what it means to become realer for a stricken but privileged portion of the population: journalists, doctors, authors, actors, academics. Since cancer and its treatments so often imperil or fracture the self, the genre of memoir—which proposes an individual identity—engages readers by evincing the resiliency of individuals who transmute or transcend their roles as patients. We need to wait and see how nonwhite and nonprofessional chroniclers will record their personal stories of cancer. But we can learn to become learners from the angry, fearful, funny, satiric, and exceptionally patient memoirists whose publications help us understand how to become our unbecoming selves.

Chapter 3

# Sublime Artistry

WHY DO GRUESOME OCCURRENCES and sights captivate us in stirring works of art? This subject has perplexed philosophers of aesthetics for centuries. That they do, however, remains indisputable. Literature thrives on miseries, conflicts, misunderstandings, blighted alternatives, and thwarted hopes. Similarly, visual artists often employ disturbing, even defiled images. In creative fiction and paintings that address the appalling consequences of disease, where might our pleasure possibly reside?

I first began thinking about the impact of startling but frightful cancer art when I looked at David Jay's photographs in *The SCAR Project* on the Web and then studied them in his 2011 book. These large-scale portraits contain images of women whose bared breasts look crumpled, concave, synthetic, reconstructed without or with reconfigured nipples, stitched horizontally or vertically or at an acute angle, lumpy, lopsided, wounded, or hacked off. I do see beauty in details: a wary smile, a cocked hat and suspenders, the branching veins of an inner arm, a mystic tattoo on a lower back, resolute hands on hips, or an abundantly pregnant belly. But in their raw engagement with mutilation, the portraits cannot be considered conventionally beautiful.

Cancer and its treatments challenge our perceptions of beauty. Without hair and breasts, some of the photographed young women had trouble feeling pretty and feminine; some felt more womanly because they realized their strength. All volunteered to participate in the project to help others confronting a cancer diagnosis and to raise awareness about the number of young adults dealing with the disease.

The valor and youthfulness of David Jay's subjects wrench me. Their bodies stopped being their own too soon. Did their selves also stop being their own too soon? Cancer scars are physical disfigurements of and on the body; but, more than that, cancer scars the psyche, the soul, the spirit. The "me" before cancer is not the "me" after cancer. Nor can the split self always be sutured. With courage, the photographed survivors bear invisible scar tissue beneath the physical scars of cancer: the haunting lost person each might have become, had it not been for the disease. They live, but not the lives they would have led.

Disturbing and yet compelling, David Jay's images trigger the mix of fright and fascination associated with the sublime. According to the philosopher Edmund Burke, whatever excites ideas of danger may become a source of the sublime, if terror is kept at some remove. Burke and his eighteenth-century contemporaries were thinking of the grandeur of the Alps or the Atlantic, when viewed from a secure but not too secure vantage. Most notably, the Romantic poets' confrontation with an overwhelming natural force threatened them with obliteration but then issued in verse of transport or exaltation. In literature, the sublime has been associated with "peak experiences" in which we apprehend or feel a force beyond the human, "a sense of something interfused that transforms a natural moment, landscape, action, or countenance."

According to the creators of the tradition traced here, a shocking and awful confrontation with an overwhelming disease also results in startling revelations, though sometimes in a less ecstatic register.

For readers or viewers, the shock and awe of the sublime are conveyed through the incongruity of "cancer art": the tension between cancer, with all its miseries, and artistry, with all its gratifications. A dreadful phenomenon brilliantly depicted may not delight but it can fascinate. "From where I sat in my cranked-up bed," Anatole Broyard explained when his prostate cancer advanced, "the sublime seemed to be all there was left."

More powerful than the beautiful, the sublime finds its source in pain and danger that pose a threat to the preservation of the individual. Of course when pain and danger press too close upon us, they cannot possibly yield ecstasy or elation but become instead simply terrible. However, representations such as David Jay's distance pain and danger sufficiently to produce in viewers or readers an awareness of the vulnerability of our being and yet also an awareness of our ability to ponder this distressing fact. The distancing we encounter in photography widens considerably in genres that we take to be not accurate records of but rather fictive responses to disease. However, such literary portrayals of cancer also attract and repulse us in the mixed states of mind that Burke's successors associated with the sublime. That we are looking at or reading about suffering in highly crafted forms reassures us that we can gain insight into the travails we ourselves may have to face.

Needless to say, I am not arguing that every work of cancer art participates in the sublime. But some of the most compelling do. At times they seem to suggest that sublimity is experienced not only by viewers and readers of representations of a dangerous, painful disease but also by sufferers of dangerous, painful diseases. Can people dying with cancer gain sufficient distance from pain to release themselves from suffering? Before and after Aleksandr Solzhenitsyn published his landmark novel *Cancer Ward* in 1967, writers have explored in their fictional accounts of terminal cancer a subjective form of time traveling that creates distance and release.

Two classic stories—Leo Tolstoy's "The Death of Ivan Ilych" and Tillie Olsen's "Tell Me a Riddle"—describe the anguish of dying from cancer, but additionally and more surprisingly they depict a mysteriously rearranged chronology that reconnects dying characters to their origins. Such transcendent moments surface without negating the cruelty of mortal suffering and the pointlessness of a death decreed by cancer. Despite our awareness of the authorial control exerted over all fictional narratives, Tolstoy and Olsen guide readers to conceive of a deathbed sublime rooted in memory and the imagination.

This difficult subject encourages me to slow down the pace, to examine Tolstoy's and Olsen's ambitious stories in some detail. I then turn to photographs, paintings, plays, novels, stories, movies, and poems in which viewers, readers, and at times characters dealing with disease experience vertiginous moments of bewildered astonishment or horrified fascination. In contrast to earlier historical periods, today illness plays a prominent role in literature, leading various authors to assert or deny the effectiveness of art as a response to disease.

In imaginative works about dying and about surviving and recovering, we will encounter portrayals of the lacerating self-hatred spawned by cancer and of compassionate caregivers who alleviate the misery of disease. But all the artists undermine the prevalent idea that patients must or can fight to win the battle against cancer. Rather, creative thinkers seek—often in experimental or shorter forms—to wrest meaning from suffering. To varying degrees, these works of art participate in an evolving cancer tradition invoking or provoking awful wonder.

Like the other creative artists discussed here, Leo Tolstoy and Tillie Olsen knew that cancer often heightens terror at the coming of death: fear of confinement in the sickroom, of the degeneration of the body, of the deathbed as torture chamber. Tolstoy's Ivan probably suffers from pancreatic cancer, Olsen's Eva from a gynecological cancer. Both characters regret who they have been (or not been) and what they have done (or not done) for and with the people closest to them. If an imminent death is the mother of regret and regret the father of anger, how can regret and anger possibly produce a sense of sublimity? In "The Death of Ivan Ilych" and "Tell Me a Riddle," terminally ill characters grapple with regret and anger before they unexpectedly experience the fearful wonder associated with the sublime.

In considering "The Death of Ivan Ilych," let's put aside Tolstoy's sarcasm about the conventionality that rules a rising class of midlevel bureaucrats, the narrator's contempt for the vanity and arrogance of his central character. What transcends satire in Tolstoy's novella is his concluding insight into pain's capacity to transform sufferers as well as his delineation throughout of a disavowal of mortality in those who attend them. A century before Philippe Ariès criticized a pervasive denial of death in *The Hour of Our Death*, Tolstoy analyzed the mechanisms whereby healthy people repudiate the reality of dying or dead human beings. Framed by the central character's funeral, the flashback that constitutes the rest of the story narrates the living and then the dying of Ivan Ilych to underscore how denial of the dying process torments the terminally ill.

After Tolstoy's protagonist hurts himself falling off a ladder while adjusting newly installed curtains (a tidy symbol of the cost of social climbing), most of those with whom he comes into contact erect a barrier between their healthy vitality and his aberrant deterioration. The doctors' indifference to the ache in his side and the queer taste in his mouth resembles his wife's efforts to evade the seriousness of his condition by emphasizing the medical routines he should be undertaking.

Besides feeling guilty about the failure of these routines or his inability to follow them or sustain faith in them, the lonely Ivan Ilych becomes encased in an all-encompassing absorption with what is wrong with his body, a lacerating and negative form of narcissism that, as a shorthand, we can call anti-narcissism: an obsession with the deteriorating self. Self-observation of "his pain and his excretions" takes up all of his attention. He can listen to others only if and when they speak about illness, hoping that their symptoms might tell him something about his own. The ongoing vigor of the living, as well as their concerted efforts to deny his condition, drives him to despair and also, even as his wife kisses his forehead, to revulsion: "he hated her from the bottom of his heart."

Although Ivan initially is locked into denial, what had screened death from him—his work schedule, his redecoration schemes—fails to hide the ache gnawing inside, the bitter taste in his mouth. The degenerating body is a relentless teacher, as he studies it in the mirror or compares his present self to portraits of his earlier self. He touches his side repeatedly, to try to convince himself that he is on the mend. But when he witnesses shock on the face of a relative who had not seen him for some time, he comes to the realization "that I'm dying, and that it's only a question of weeks, days. . . ."

Sheer terror of the unnamable is his first response to death: "*It* drew his attention to itself . . . only so that he should look at *It*, look *It* straight in the face: look at *It* and without doing anything, suffer inexpressibly." Constricted within a dulling depression, he suffers the misery of special arrangements having to be made for his excretions—"a torment from the uncleanliness, the unseemliness, and the smell, and from knowing that another person had to take part in it"—and also the lie "that he was not dying but was simply ill." Toward the end, powerful opiates fail to relieve Ivan Ilych's physical anguish and psychological isolation. Screaming for three days, he protests his pain and his incomprehension of it. Ivan struggles with the agony of being thrust into what Tolstoy describes as a black bag or sack until he finally achieves an unanticipated breakthrough.

In my early teaching days, I interpreted Ivan's deathbed judgment—"it was all not the right thing"—as a condemnation of the moral shambles of his life, a discernment that then enables him to see the light. But this does not accurately capture the sequence of events as they appear on the page. First, "some force struck him in the chest and side, making it even harder to breathe, and *he fell through the hole* and there at the bottom was a light" (emphasis mine). A painful and random blow leads to release, as if the dynamics of prolonged pain thrust the sufferer into another realm.

How very curious that there is an additional account of how Ivan gets out of the black bag, quite inconsistent with the first. After we are informed that "some force" released Ivan, we learn that Ivan's son had come to his bedside and caught his hand "and began to cry": "*At that very moment*, Ivan Ilych *fell through* and caught sight of the light, and it was revealed to him that though his life had not been what it should have been, it could still be rectified" (emphasis mine). In the first telling, release from suffering is as chancy and aimless as his original injury; but in the second, the tears of a compassionate witness liberate Ivan from his confinement, just as earlier he had understood his fate by seeing the shock on a relative's face.

When in the second telling Ivan's son sidesteps all the falsity to witness his father's misery, the dying man perceives the anguish of his survivors, and this interpersonal witnessing—the son weeping for his father, the father grieving for his son and then his wife— ruptures pain's carapace. At the end of his life, Ivan Ilych does not think, "Life is finished." Instead, he exclaims, "Death is finished . . . it is no more."

No longer capitalized as "*It*," death, he finally realizes, does not constitute the end of everything. Previously, Ivan Ilych had thought, "When I am not, what will there be? There will be nothing." But now he passes beyond hatred and torment, forgoing life, forgiving death, for the extinguishing of his individual being does not stop existence in general or the survival of his family in particular. The last words Ivan Ilych speaks on his deathbed are "What joy!" After great pain, such unanticipated joy returns us to the puzzling contradiction between the two accounts of release from the black sack. They might, of course, bespeak a tug-of-war within Tolstoy between his aesthetic commitment (to recording the dynamics of prolonged pain) and his ethical motive (to use fiction to teach the efficacy of empathy).

But can the inconsistency also be identified with incoherence during the last stages of consciousness? Being pushed through the black bag of dying prompts responses similar to those apparent in the newly born: dazed sleepiness, extreme weakness, incomprehensible cries, flailing limbs, startling, difficulty breathing. "Death labors" is the term used by one critic for this phenomenon. According to E. M. Forster, "the memory of birth and the expectation of death always lurk within the human being. . . . Naked I came into the world, naked I shall go out of it." For beings at the beginning and the ending of life, it seems, the dimensions of the universe contract and expand in ways that those of us in the middle passage cannot fully comprehend. "The Death of Ivan Ilych" illuminates the idea that "death's delirium loosens the links of linearity," thereby allowing "life's moments to regroup themselves according to alternative priorities" urgently needed by the person dying.

The zigzagging or interweaving tracks of time in the terminal condition explain the two contradictory accounts of Ivan's release from the black bag two hours before his death. What I took to be a glitch reflects bewildering uncertainties attendant on the dying— or, to be more exact, a circling back or crisscrossing of consciousness as a series of frozen frames come into view. Whether the force preceded the boy or was initiated by the boy is a discrimination that one cannot make in a hallucinatory state.

A fascinating analogy, suggesting that space shifts for the dying person, appears between the two tellings: "What had happened to him was like the sensation one sometimes experiences in a railway carriage when one thinks one is going backwards while one is really going forwards and suddenly becomes aware of the real direction." This spatial perplexity mirrors Ivan's earlier temporal bewilderment, his concentration on his progression forward toward death during weeks that have repeatedly sent him back in time to memories of "all the joys, griefs, and delights of childhood, boyhood, and youth."

During his suffering and despite his graying beard, Ivan Ilych had wanted "someone to pity him as a sick child is pitied." The first feeling of being thrust into a deep black sack produced helplessness, and he wept "like a child." As he declines into infantile dependence, it begins to dawn on him that only in childhood had there been "something really pleasant," and his professional ascent has in fact been a descent from the delights he had known in his youth: "It is as if I had been going downhill while I imagined I was going up." When he becomes too frail to leave the sofa, vivid memories of the past resurface. Because "There's one bright spot there at the back, at the beginning of life," as his future disappears he speeds back toward his origins.

The temporal and spatial confusion between up and down, back and forward, end and beginning reminds us that the novella opens with a death notice in the daily newspaper and a meeting of friends under a clock. On his deathbed, Ivan is dislocated from the temporal frame of daily newspapers and clocks. During his three days of continued screaming, we are told, "time did not exist for him." His final words of joy are followed by the narrator's attention to the strange temporality of the dying: "To him all this happened in a single instant, and the meaning of that instant did not change. For those present his agony continued for another two hours."

During his dying, Ivan is removed and elsewhere—passing out of the body bag into the light. Not Elisabeth Kübler-Ross's final stage of acceptance but rather immutable joy permeates the eternal instant of Ivan Ilych's last moment of consciousness during the concluding hours of his demise. Generations of readers have been baffled and moved by his howling, joyous death.

Like Tolstoy's story, Tillie Olsen's "Tell Me a Riddle" suggests that the sublime liberates the dying from the death toward which they career. Even before a cancer diagnosis, Eva's anger spills over into resentment of her spouse in a way that recalls the hostility of Tolstoy's protagonist. Unlike Ivan, though, Eva fulminates against the domestic and economic privations she suffered as an impoverished immigrant. The story takes on extraordinary poignancy when the aging Eva—unnamed until the final pages of the tale—realizes that maternal and wifely duties have obscured the fervent convictions of her youthful self. As she lies dying of cancer, Eva gives voice to the survival, against great odds, of a passionate vision of social justice that she accesses through her terminal time traveling. Although "Tell Me a Riddle" revolves around a character who resists searching for her buried self or, indeed, journeying anywhere, Eva will find herself traveling incessantly through time and space.

Before her cancer is diagnosed, disease puts Eva back in contact with memories of herself as an overworked mother of seven children and as a destitute girl in a Russian village. While she and her husband, David, battle over selling their house, however, Eva does not know what ails her: "She did not know if the tumult was outside or in her. Always a ravening inside, a pull to the bed, to lie down, to succumb." The first section of "Tell Me a Riddle" concludes with a chorus of Eva's adult children. What they took to be a psychosomatic manifestation of her bitterness was "cancer . . . everywhere, surrounding the liver, everywhere," a diagnosis they withhold from her.

After an operation, Eva fulminates at having been put on a list of Jewish patients to be visited by a rabbi in the hospital: outraged, she wishes to declare "Race, human; Religion, none." Embracing the secular humanism of her youth—her husband David taunts, "You think you are still an orator of the 1905 revolution?"—Eva wants "To smash all ghettos that still divide us." As her family forces Eva to journey westward to visit her adult children, she travels eastward into the Russian past.

Because sickness incapacitates Eva, guilt about maternal inadequacy is the form taken by anti-narcissism in "Tell Me a Riddle." While the passion of tending her own babies "had risen with the need like a torrent," in Ohio she cannot bear holding her newborn grandchild, who brings back "warm flesh" that "nuzzled away all else with lovely mouths devoured." Post-operative fatigue and unacknowledged disease render her unable to save her daughter from the riddle of maternity, from "drowning into needing and being needed." Feeling useless, desperately wanting to go home, riddled by disease that has made her "all bones and a swollen belly," she must submit to visiting her other children in California.

At a turning point in the third section, Eva's memories of Russia begin to transform her, in David's teasing appellations, from Mrs. Word Miser to Mrs. Orator-without-Breath. She encounters various relatives who spark recollections of her youth. The clash between the idealism of Russia fifty years ago and the materialism of America in the fifties comes to a head at a concert, with the result that Eva, overcome by dizziness, dwindles into a gagging "swollen thinness." A cacophony of chants, croons, serenades, and songs brings back a memory of her childhood self—"*a bare footed sore-covered little girl*" dancing "*her ecstasy of grimace*" at a village wedding. She then puzzles over a dream deferred while gasping and sobbing for breath.

Unable to reconcile decades of violence and her earlier belief in the progress of humankind, Eva appeals to her husband, "Man . . . we'll destroy ourselves?" At that moment she sees "the helpless pity and fear for her (for *her*)" in David's face and realizes she is dying. As in Tolstoy's tale, a compassionate witness pierces the fog of lies.

When Eva takes to her deathbed in a West Coast apartment with David, their granddaughter Jeannie reminds the feverish Eva of a girl named Lisa who first taught Eva that "life was holy, knowledge was holy." Through phrases fractured by pain and fatigue, we come to understand that Lisa was hanged for killing someone who had betrayed many, committing the murder before Eva's eyes when they were both political prisoners. Early on, then, Eva reveled in a courageous commitment to social justice, even as she witnessed the anarchic nihilism of politics. As infusions are administered and Eva grows lighter "like a bird," her incoherent phrases some-times mention atrocities—"*Slaveships deathtrains*"—sometimes protests against atrocities: "*No man one except through others.*" Her delirium profoundly hurts her husband, for she recalls "nothing of him, of the children, of their intimate life together." Despite her husband's taunts at her orations clamoring for justice and freedom, he remembers with "shame . . . a girl's voice of eloquence that spoke their holiest dreams."

Eva's singing of the socialist hymn "These Things Shall Be" while David plunks down cards from a solitaire deck finally punc-tures his defensive denials even as it expresses a political impasse experienced by many. Her hopes for a regenerated human race—"*They shall be gentle, brave and strong / to spill no drop of blood, but dare / all . . .*"—shock David out of hooting at the cadaver's belief that ignorance and prejudice will evaporate in the twentieth cen-tury. During her dying, Eva confronts her abiding idealism in the perfectibility of humankind and her alarm at repeated challenges to that faith.

The last paragraph of "Tell Me a Riddle" describes Eva's death-bed agony and David's desire to flee until Jeannie comforts him with her grandmother's promise: "On the last day, she said she would go back to when she first heard music," to a wedding at which "they dance, while the flutes so joyous and vibrant tremble in the air." But Jeannie's story prettifies Eva's earlier memory of the wedding—the "*sore-covered*" girl dancing "*her ecstasy of grimace to the flutes that scratched.*" Jeannie glosses over the fervent aspirations and miserable disappointments of Eva's abiding commitment to a lost cause.

Through the broken singing of "These Things Shall Be," Eva grapples with one of the many riddles addressed by the story. What transports us beyond our individual selves is an uplifting ideal of continual engagement in the struggle for social justice; what terrifies is the prospect that this ideal has been overwhelmed by the accumulated and accumulating nightmares of history. Through Eva's deathbed aria, Olsen grapples with the ultimate riddle addressed by the story: how is it that the process of dying may return us to who we were when we became ourselves?

Like Tolstoy, Olsen uses terminal cancer to posit the idea that in our end is our beginning. To some extent, of course, their characters' fates reflect the need of creative writers to arrive at a fulfilling conclusion. Yet both authors believe that dying people become quixotic time travelers. Fueled by memories and songs, imaginative time travel appears to be triggered by the ghastly anti-narcissism that accompanies the dying—but this time travel also alleviates anti-narcissism.

Though it takes many forms, obsessive loathing of the diseased body, together with stymied or twisted familial love, contributes to the cognitive exhaustion and bafflement of characters who nevertheless end up glimpsing an integrity of self that cannot be rationally comprehended by themselves or communicated to others. Does the failure of the body, the mind, and the senses precede a subjective flooding of compensatory imaginings? Such deathbed sublimity might seem improbable, but after exhaustion and pain have made regret, anger, and all physical and mental exertions futile, perhaps imaginative forms of apprehension arise. Using quite different formal techniques, Tolstoy affirms the final words of Olsen's story: *"Death deepens the wonder."*

According to Tolstoy and Olsen, deathbed wanderings—for the most part opaque to survivors—turn the attention of the dying away from their imminent annihilation and transform them from victims to seers. Sublime encounters insulate and shield the dying person from the dying process, from the ghastly physical agonies witnessed by caregivers. This disjunction transforms the dying into resident aliens—at least in fiction. Tolstoy and Olsen revise one of the most famous maxims about death, Epicurus's pronouncement that we are not present at it. Their stories suggest that where the dying are, death is not; where death is, the living are. Relieved for Ivan and Eva, I suspect that I, too, wouldn't mind being elsewhere when the great event occurs.

But even in fiction, the legitimacy of the deathbed sublime is left indeterminate. Ivan's confusion and Eva's fragmented communications qualify our knowledge of them. So if there is a sublime subject, it resides less in the dying central characters than in the living readers of these stories. While reading, we recognize, on the one hand, the horrible corruption of the diseased body and, on the other, the wondrous exaltation of release from it. Within the story (for its central character) and outside the story (for interpreters), the peak experience of the sublime arises from the imagination confronting its imminent dissolution. In response to death, which cannot be represented, the imagination of characters and their authors proposes disjointed images and associations that awe us with our need to comprehend the incomprehensible.

Provoking us to feel for and with characters dealing with terminal disease, the sublime plays a role not only in fiction about death but also in visual art about cancer treatment. In viewing photographs and paintings, however, we never gain even the limited sort of access to subjectivity that Tolstoy and Olsen give us into Ivan's and Eva's thoughts and emotions. Instead, our tangled fascination and aversion derive from the weird juxtaposition between content—the patient's lack of control—and form: the artist's command, exerted primarily through cultural references. The detached scene of treatment within a framed photographed or painted image raises a host of unanswerable questions about the specifics of the individual's background, of diagnosis and prognosis—information withheld from us. What we are given, instead, is the larger cultural context furnished by allusions.

When Hannah Wilke and Robert Pope put on display their own or another person's suffering, they cross a line of privacy that most of us respect, and their transgression renders their work unsettling. They do so to propose a genealogy of suffering that makes the experiences of cancer patients less anomalous, though perhaps more disturbing.

Hannah Wilke was accused of narcissistic display when she produced photographs of body performances in the 1970s and '80s, but in her later series *Intra-Venus* she explores the anti-narcissism prompted by intravenous treatments for leukemia. Scenes generally hidden from view—concealed inside hospitals and behind privacy curtains—become a spectacle involving a body stripped not only of clothing but even of a flimsy hospital gown.

On the Web, you can find Wilke's images of herself as a sick, naked patient with bloodied body bandages on both hips, or bloated in a bed with tubes infusing the chemotherapy that caused her weight gain, or sitting on a plastic commode, again attached to infusion equipment. These pictures cannot but instill fear at the fatigue evident in the downward cast and shadowed eyes, the flaccid flesh, the hair loss. To some, they may look repugnant, perhaps even masochistic or sensational. Yet because Wilke orchestrated the staging and the taking of these visceral photographs, we understand her to be not only the model but also the creator, not just an object but also a subject.

In this regard, the series *Intra-Venus* differs from the series of paintings Ferdinand Hodler produced from 1905 to 1915 of his dying model, Valentine Gode-Darel, who, after two breast surgeries, deteriorates from a vertical strong young woman to a horizontal debased corpse. Touching as some of these images are, it is impossible not to think about the artist drawing while his model is dying, his making something permanent of the absence she will become. To this extent, the paintings seem exploitative.

But Wilke actively directed her husband, Donald Goddard, to produce lasting images out of her passivity as a patient and her impending erasure. Her agency is revealed through her allusions to cultural history. So, for example, the image of her washing herself in a shower is taken through a shower curtain and recalls the frightful murder in *Psycho*. Her most famous photograph of herself wrapped in a blue hospital blanket invokes Titian's *Mater Doloroso*, the Mother of Sorrows. When she balances a vase of flowers on her head, it is impossible not to think of William Tell or, for that matter, William Burroughs, who balanced an apple on his wife's head and then shot her.

Such references to iconic women—murdered or burdened—indicate how staged and symbolic the artist's undertaking remains. Wilke's deliberately designed allusions contrast with all that is beyond her control: the IVs, bandages, incisions at the lymph nodes in her neck, thinning pubic hair. Her commanding photographs stop the flow of time, preserving one singular and staged moment from mutability.

So do the paintings of Robert Pope, who made cancer treatment his subject and emphasized the artifice of his work by invoking cultural iconography, in his case the iconography of Christianity. A few years before he died of Hodgkin's disease in 1992, Pope created evocative works about the fraught experiences of the patients he saw during a succession of hospitalizations. Social realism meets surrealism in large canvases that portray the loneliness of sick men and women within the sterility of contemporary hospitals. Pope's works—reproduced in the book *Illness & Healing*—conflate modern medicine with archaic rituals of blood sacrifice. They unsettle viewers because his human figures reenact primitive, fearful rites in technologically advanced settings.

In *Radiation*, for example, a man lies alone on a narrow plank beneath a huge machine directing rays at his abdomen. Pope explains that "the red lasers which are used for positioning suggest a Christian cross, the table the man lies on is like an altar, he is covered with a white shroud, the machine hovers above him like an idol or faceless god that must be propitiated with bodily sacrifices." In a scene straight out of science fiction, the patient holds still in a black void. A marked man, he is caught in the beamed crosshairs, exposing himself to a dreaded otherness that he cannot possibly understand and that all others flee. He, like the viewer, must wonder whether its invisible powers will heal or harm him. The artist emphasizes the mysterious medical protocols to which patients submit even though they cannot rationally comprehend them.

Another acrylic painting, *Chemotherapy*, presents a turbaned woman lying on her side and pulling up a sheet to cover herself. Beneath her, in the foreground, a disproportionately large syringe of Adriamycin looms. The chemical is red, like life-giving blood and the Red Cross, but also like an alarming stop sign or an inferno (it is nicknamed the "red devil"). The knot on her turban parallels the knot of her clenched knuckles, all imbued with the pigment called "caput mortuum" (literally, "dead head"), which is the color of dried blood. Does the patient shrink from a drug that will debilitate her, or does she welcome its curative capacities? Does she want to shield herself with the sheet, or shroud herself? In contrast to the specificity of Hannah Wilke's photographs of herself, the nameless woman painted by Pope could be anyone or a composite of several people. Does the unrealistically enlarged syringe at the bottom of the painting replace her signature? Will the drug erase her individuality by turning her into a sort of replicant of herself?

In paintings with other figures, the perspective generally remains that of the patient in the hospital bed—again prone, but sometimes without a head. For we view the scene from the patient's perspective, as if we were he. From his vantage, white-coated physicians tower over him, as do most visitors. In a self-portrait with Robert Pope's doctor, the physical closeness between the standing physician and the seated patient is meant to convey the relationship between "priest and layperson." Next to a bedside picture of Jesus in another work, Pope draws a tray of syringes to suggest that "faith in science has replaced faith in religion." Like most religions, the religion of cancer treatments involves mysterious rituals undertaken by those hopeful for salvation but also fearful of punishment.

Even when Pope's figures are upright and vertical and entwined, they are riven on the stake. In the 6-foot-high *Hug*, the embracing patient and caregiver are divided—here by the IV rod that sunders the couple "like a dagger," in the artist's words. Although the man and woman encircle each other, they are cleaved by the cross of the IV pole, holding high its bag of solutions. The intravenous tubes twisting around the pole form the spiral figure of infinity, but in some drafts the tubes look serpentine.

If we see the IV pole as encircled by snakes, we will recall the rod of Asclepius, the classical god of healing and medicine. The frequent confusion of the rod of Asclepius with Hermes' caduceus is telling, for Hermes' staff is associated with commerce. Are the embracing man and woman entangled in the big business of medicine, or are they entwined in the healing arts? Will the loving couple be destroyed by venomous toxins, or sustained in the continuum of life and death? In the cancer dance, the melding patient and caregiver look indistinguishable. Though the female figure is barefoot and must be the patient, both huggers are entangled in the paraphernalia of treatment.

The visual arts encourage us to study physical surfaces instead of psychological depths, which seems appropriate. According to both Wilke and Pope, patients cannot possibly fathom what will result from treatment. Wilke's photographs and Pope's paintings evoke fear as well as awe: fear at what powerful medical technologies do to people's bodies, awe that patients find the fortitude to submit to them. Some viewers may also feel guilt or perplexity at scrutinizing people repeatedly probed and scanned.

While putting the visible effects of treatment in the context not of a personal history but of a larger cultural framework, the images of Wilke and Pope pull back the privacy curtain. I am more discomforted by the photographs of Wilke than by Pope's portraits of patients, yet both repudiate the denial of dying so passionately criticized by Tolstoy. In the process, they transform cancer treatments from a shameful secret into an experience of a piece with the sorrowful human condition.

The sublime springs from a fearful awareness that disease bequeaths: an intuition that the future is radically abridged shockingly saturates the present with mortality. Here at the very start of my day, in the middle of my mundane life, looms the end. If we want to understand the consequences of this buckling of time, we must return to the writers preoccupied by the imminent endings of cancer stories. Just as patients are haunted after prognosis by statistical approximations of their death, the opening scenes in fiction about cancer are often shadowed by the anticipation of closing scenes. Such poignant foreknowledge can produce melodramatic tearjerkers, but it also teases writers to test the utility of art: if we know the end of the story from the start, why should we bother to read or watch it?

Writers tackling this question have proved that the aesthetic landscape has changed since the early twentieth century. In contrast to the paucity of imaginative books about sickness decried by Virginia Woolf in *On Being Ill,* creative works about cancer proliferate today, and the more intriguing among them encourage us to contemplate their own efficacy, to gauge what difference they make in terms of suffering that remains intractable and inexorable.

In one case, a playwright has produced a qualified defense of reading, associating it with caregiving that ameliorates the frightfulness of late-stage disease. For many novelists as well, the figure of the caregiver tempers the terrors of cancer and its treatment and in so doing provides needed distance from them. Although nothing can be done to rescue the dying from death, the attendance of the caregiver—and often, too, the caregiver's engagement with reading or writing—effectively delivers a precious gift: the gift of staying attached to and bonded with the dying, and thereby preserving a remnant of their humanity until the end.

Margaret Edson's unsettling play *Wit* censures the power invested in scientific and humanistic forms of knowledge. "My treatment imperils my health," the main character exclaims about harsh medical protocols, but the same claim can be made about the values by which she has lived. A punctilious English professor who obsesses over the commas and periods in John Donne's sonnets, Vivian Bearing has only one visitor during a lengthy hospitalization for experimental chemotherapy. She remains as isolated in the hospital as she had been in her life. The intellect she prizes in poetry cannot save her from the intellect of the doctors who reduce her to a text, a specimen to be endlessly manipulated. Depersonalized by clinicians, humiliated by invasive procedures, depleted by drugs, and written up in research reports, Vivian Bearing bears the suffering of terminal medical technologies. Yet during her professional career she had dedicated herself to a highly specialized expertise related, like the doctors', to interpreting little black marks on pieces of paper.

Only during her dying does Vivian discover that compassion remains the fundamental that both she and her doctors had scorned but now need. At this point in the play, moralism begins to tame the sublime. The cerebral academic receives words of wisdom from her caring nurse and from a visiting teacher, a great-grandmother who cradles her while reading aloud Margaret Wise Brown's *The Runaway Bunny*, a children's book about an all-caring mother: "'If you become a bird and fly away from me,' said his mother, 'I will be a tree that you come home to.'" The elderly mentor interprets the story as "a little allegory of the soul. No matter where it hides, God will find it." *Wit* here leads the audience to suppose that the emotive power of literature may be less suspect than the manipulative powers of scientific and humanistic knowledge. Finally after her death, Vivian arises naked—to reach toward a stage light—suggesting that she now understands death not as a final period but as a tentative comma leading to another phase of existence.

*Wit* transcends its own didacticism in the thrilling theatricality of its ending and also in the allegorically named character's repeated asides: "if you think eight months of cancer treatment is tedious for the *audience*, consider how it feels to play the part." The jarring idea of going out to a "show" or settling down to "an entertaining feature" about degeneration and death underscores the incongruity of combining art, associated with pleasure, and cancer, associated with pain. This dissonance is repeatedly conjured in a number of novels that use cancer to investigate the usefulness of narration when we know the finish at the start. Exploring cancer's deformation of time and the anti-narcissism of the dying, their authors stake out a claim for narrative's worth by emphasizing the crucial role played by compassionate witnessing.

In three representative novels, as in *Wit*, the figure of the caregiver—whose empathy alleviates the horror of disease for the dying—mitigates the terror of terminal cancer for the reader. Not necessarily understanding what is witnessed, the caregiver nevertheless remains present to and with the dying, connected even during the incomprehensible moment when being transmogrifies into non-being. The character of the compassionate witness serves as a model for the novelists and for their task.

J. M. Coetzee's *Age of Iron* consists of an extended letter composed by an elderly woman dying of breast cancer, who describes the horrors of South African apartheid to her daughter in America. Like Solzhenitsyn, who identified cancer with the malignant growth of Stalin's labor camps, Coetzee's Mrs. Curren links her cancer with a diseased body politic, an apartheid system based on white liberals' collusion with the brutality of genocide. "I have cancer from the accumulation of shame I have endured in my life. That is how cancer comes about: from self-loathing the body turns malignant and begins to eat away at itself."

Seeing the police destroying a black township, Mrs. Curren equates the "monstrous growths" of cancer with "misbirths": a sign that one is "beyond one's term." Having "fallen pregnant with these growths, these cold, obscene swellings; to have carried and carried this brood beyond any natural term, unable to bear them, unable to sate their hunger," she must make ready for the end so something can arise from the ashes, as should her country. According to Coetzee, apartheid will issue only in death. Similarly, Mrs. Curren has "a child inside that I cannot give birth to": "So it is my prisoner or I am its prisoner. It beats on the gate but it cannot leave."

For most of Mrs. Curren's letter, she believes that she is addressing her daughter "as the beloved, as that which does not die": "It is the soul of you that I address, as it is the soul of me that will be left with you when this letter is over." And so she describes her struggle with ineffective drugs, her aches and pains, her vacillations and ramblings, as she shakes "loose from the dying envelope." A drunken homeless man whom she has taken into her house has promised to mail the letter after her death.

Toward the end of her epistolary narrative, he starts to become not merely the messenger but also the mystic message, a sort of "angel come to show me the way." Watching over her, washing her underclothes, and witnessing her pain, this most unlikely of caregivers—a homeless angel of death—becomes a new beloved who unlooses her from her beleaguered body through an embrace from which "there was no warmth to be had." That he is neither the recipient nor the intended reader of her prose account underscores the uncanny nature of their bond.

The concept of the sublime is directly addressed by a caregiver in Andrew Solomon's autobiographical novel *A Stone Boat*. The youthful narrator, Harry, a classical pianist, confronts the extended dying of his charismatic mother with the realization that "the sublime is a matter of exchanging easier for more difficult pleasures." Harry does not choose to relinquish the easy pleasures of his early intimacy with his adoring mother. Her ovarian cancer forces him to do so, for she becomes furious at herself, at the luxurious world from which the disease cuts her off, and also at her son, blaming the diagnosis on her anguish over his homosexuality: "my disease was killing her and would kill her." As Harry crisscrosses the Atlantic, engaging in a series of erotic relationships, his mother—engulfed in depression—"hated her doctors, and she hated the hospital, and she hated her treatments, and she hated all the disciplined isolation."

Harry, together with his brother and his father, eventually joins his mother in revulsion at the "glowing enthusiastic optimistic vocabulary" of "butterscotch" doctors who subject the once beautiful woman to debilitating and pointless treatments. As his mother begins to come to terms with Harry's sexuality, his coming-of-age story is overtaken by her quest for a dignified death. Determined to gain the assistance of her husband and sons in helping her to die, she has them study "a booklet for people who want to end their own lives"; they need to do it right "for legal and medical reasons." She then orchestrates a deathbed scene "as grand and rich, as well-conceived and as stunning as *La Traviata*'s." Solomon depicts the pained reactions of family members as they help her kill herself, for he wants to capture the emotional complexity of a planned death.

All the mother's rage and despair evaporate once she has regained some control through the pills she has stashed away. Her deeply appreciative deathbed words shape Harry's final vision of her, which, in turn, empowers him to speak and write about her and his love of her. Yet, as Solomon also explains in a number of nonfictional works, the liberation accomplished by an assisted suicide takes a heavy toll on caregivers, who feel complicit in a murder. Glittering with precious jewels, the stone boat of his novel's title may be "breathtaking to watch," but it does not float.

Redemptive caregiving pervades the graphic novel *When David Lost His Voice*, which experiments with all sorts of visual forms to consider how anxiety about cancer metastasizes in a family. The

Belgian author and illustrator Judith Vanistendael employs impressionist paintings, watercolors, pen-and-ink sketches, pastel children's book illustrations, the anatomical diagrams that doctors draw for patients, surrealistic dream landscapes, film clips, and black-and-white murals. The narrative focuses on the women in David's life while he deals with treatments for the larynx cancer that will kill him. A succession of pictures recount the resourceful ways in which loving relatives deal with illness and with the silence spawned by a patient's dread of disease and death.

A conflation of ends and beginnings, death and life, opens the book, for the shock of diagnosis is followed by a dream sequence in which first David receives "a lucky charm" of "divine light" from his childhood nanny and then a granddaughter emerges from the swirling waters of the birth canal of David's older daughter, Miriam. An especially resonant series of frames later illuminates Miriam's fear of her father's imminent mortality. In a bookstore, she hallucinates seeing him as a skeleton; his flesh dissolves to reveal his skull and then returns to restore his face.

Arrivals and departures also haunt David's artist-wife, Paula, who suffers from his reticence while using her art to deal with her distress about scans. After Paula escapes David's silence to give a lecture in Helsinki, a series of very dark pictures depict her encounter with a stranger who rescues her from freezing on a boat stuck in ice: "I'm giving you a boat that stops time!" she yells at her absent husband. Three vertical frames on one page slow down time as the stranger embraces her and she thanks him for his smell, because the chemo has changed her husband's characteristic scent.

Much brighter and gayer in color are those portions of the book devoted to Paula and David's relationship with their 9-year-old daughter, Tamar. For example, in one section both parents collude in her fantasy that letters can be delivered via balloons. Pictures of Tamar's last boat trip with David, her swim with the mermaid friend she finds in the sea, and her conversations with a real friend about how to preserve her father's soul in a jar, as well as drawings of her bathing with her father and lying with him in his sickbed: these beautiful images depict the child's fear of abandonment and her imaginative means of sustaining a loving relationship with him.

In the hospital, when she hugs his emaciated body after his larynx has been removed, Tamar asks him to "Stay with me. . . . ." Unable to speak, David writes her a note, "My darling, I am with you," which she puts in a vial and strings around her neck. Before and after this gift of a fragile textual totem, *When David Lost His Voice* squarely confronts the end-of-life desolation and hallucinations brought about by hospitalization and morphine, raising difficult moral questions about operations performed to preserve the lives of people who no longer want them and about the responsibility of doctors who are asked to help those people die.

Although we know at the start how these novels will end, they draw us into imagined communities that confront and crystallize some of the ethical and psychological dilemmas posed by cancer. And through the characters of a homeless angel, a loving son who helps his mother kill herself, and a child finding creative ways to stay attached to her dying father, we identify with acts and sentiments of empathy that in turn create sympathy in us for those undergoing the degeneration of a mortal disease. The authors of these caregiving characters endorse the value of narration in consolidating human bonds while accepting that it is futile in staunching suffering or staving off death. They thereby serve as compassionate witnesses of compassionate witnesses.

It would be too much to expect the edgy sublime to inform a commercially successful television series about cancer patients. Yet it does play a major role in the cascading violence of *Breaking Bad*. The malevolence of cancer as well as the terror and rage it can spawn infiltrates this gripping television series from start to finish. Not only is the central character motivated to make crystal meth to pay for his treatment, but cancer also represents the malignant nihilism that has turned Walt Whitman's America into the brutal society inhabited by an increasingly brutal Walt White.

Of course most movies about cancer—from *Love Story* and *Brian's Song* to *Matching Jack* and *50/50*—are properly classified as "inspirational." But a few address the shock and awe of diagnosis and treatment. The Japanese film *Ikuru*, inspired by "The Death of Ivan Ilych," captures the terror of its protagonist as a cancer diagnosis transforms his timid life into an experiment in societal giving. *One True Thing* (an adaptation of the novel by Anna Quindlen), *My Life without Me* (an adaptation of a story by Nanci Kincaid), and *Southern Comfort*, all dealing with ovarian cancer, implicitly question cheerful recovery stories by addressing terminal disease.

Perhaps shorter forms, such as television episodes of *Breaking Bad* and also of *The Big C*, can more easily sustain the intensity of the sublime. Beginning with Tolstoy, the short story plays a large role in the cancer canon. "Tell me things I won't mind forgetting," the dying character says in Amy Hempel's story "In the Cemetery Where Al Jolson Is Buried." And much of the story consists of the stories her best friend tells as they sit—like "Lucy and Ethel, Mary and Rhoda in extremis"—on hospital beds. Why are we often given cancer stories about story-telling?

Stories about stories enable fiction writers to engage the terms "cancer" and "art" and contemplate their relation; but brilliant practitioners of the genre arrive at strikingly dissimilar perspectives. Alice Munro emphasizes the paradoxical liberations of cancer and art, while Lorrie Moore deplores their pernicious perils. Personally, I would rather inhabit Alice Munro's fictional landscapes, fraught though they can be. But it is Lorrie Moore who makes the hairs on my arms stand up. For this reason, I will conclude this discussion of fiction with the works of Munro and Moore, before briefly glancing at the minimalist form of the lyric in which contemporary poets mine the present tense to express the alarm that startles people from the moment of cancer's detection throughout their subsequent efforts to deal with the disease.

Two stories about cancer by Alice Munro ignite and then defuse the reader's fear of potential violence against women. At the start of "Floating Bridge," Munro explores the ironic freedom bequeathed by a cancer that the central character previously assumed to be terminal. Living in a desolate town with a feckless hippy husband, Jinny must have seen her impending death as an opportunity to escape all the dingy compromises and petty resentments of her life, for the good news delivered by her "cautiously optimistic" oncologist "made everything harder"—so much harder that Jinny refrains from sharing it with anyone. Even the reader does not realize that she is in remission until more than halfway through the story.

Munro captures the unanticipated distress of remission, which can rob a patient like Jinny of "a certain low-grade freedom." The reprieve means that she must confront what she now knows to be an unsatisfactory marriage: it was as if a "dull, protecting membrane . . . had been pulled away and left her raw." These thoughts occur to her as a lout tells her a dirty joke. That the story's punch line involves a father and son's hunt for "pussy" underscores the bankruptcy of Jinny's relationship with her philandering husband and adds a sinister twist to the appearance of the joke teller's teenage son, Ricky, who offers to drive her home.

As the sun sets, Ricky takes a deserted road, explaining that he won't turn the car lights on until they can see the stars. Jinny realizes they have stopped on a bridge "of crossways-laid planks. No railings. And motionless water underneath it." While she thinks, "This is where he brings his girls," she realizes that before diagnosis she would have been frightened. A mile further on, he tells her to "walk a ways with me," an ominous instruction in this remote setting. Their footsteps turn the boards beneath their feet into the rising and falling deck of a boat. Looking down on the side, they see "stars riding on the water." After Ricky kisses Jinny on the mouth, the story ends with her unexpected elation in this precarious moment: "What she felt was a lighthearted sort of compassion, almost like laughter. A swish of tender hilarity, getting the better of all her sores and hollows, for the time given." Jinny loses her unease, momentarily accepting the new experience and the instability it entails.

The transformation of time initiated by prognosis may free a patient not just to assess what is wrong with the life she has been living but also to take risks. Because remission brings to mind recurrence, a cancer survivor quoted in Musa Mayer's *After Breast Cancer* repeats an oncologist's response to her fears: "Once you've had cancer you spend the rest of your life on a rickety bridge." Ricky cannot be considered a reliable friend who will comfort Jinny or take her part when darkness falls and pain is all around. What eases her is not a sturdy bridge over troubled waters but a precarious floating bridge. And yet in the "swish" of the ephemeral, she shines.

Living with cancer, according to Munro, involves acknowledging the unpredictability of ever-shifting notions of the length of one's own future and equally fluctuating emotional responses to a radically foreshortened or lengthened life expectancy. Such a hallucinogenic future imbues the present moment with the mystic resonance to which many patients attest when they talk about cancer granting them a realization of the preciousness of existence.

Munro's second story about cancer, "Free Radicals," also fuels growing apprehension that a strange man will assault a sick woman in a desolate place, and its conclusion also reverses this expectation. In a curious way, the plot hints that cancer is experienced as an interloper, a malevolent intruder who terrifies the occupant of the house. Before an actual maniac appears, however, Nita had been dealing with the shock of her healthy 81-year-old husband's sudden death as well as the malignant growths on her liver, diminished but not gone for good.

Residing in the house her husband had built for his first wife, Nita is so disabled by grief and by drugs that she finds herself unable to read, even though she loved reading before: "Always fiction. She hated to hear the word 'escape' used about fiction." On a hot summer day, a young man appears, looking "more wasted than boyish." When he smashes a plate on the floor and scrapes a shard down his forearm to produce beads of blood, it becomes clear that her life is in danger. Having to deal with cancer does not stop other terrible events from occuring.

Like Nita's love of reading, the intruder's macabre tale alerts us to the thematic importance of narrative. The anonymous stranger wants to tell Nita a story about a photograph of an old couple sitting on a couch and a large younger woman in a wheelchair nearby: his father, mother, and the older sister who "just set out to torment me," he says. His tale involves a family reunion at which he snapped the photo and then shot all three. An "after" photo shows their expressions "blown away." By this time, Nita's legs are shaking and a terminal diagnosis is no help: "The fact that she was going to die within a year refused to cancel out the fact that she might die now." She protects herself against the psychopath's narrative by offering one of her own. Over the drink he demands, Nita hazards a guess that he had never killed before and then states that she, like he, has murdered, in her case using poison to dispatch "the girl my husband was in love with." The tale is fabricated out of what she suspects must have been the anger directed at her by her husband's first wife.

Within the context of the story's title—an allusion to highly reactive and unstable atoms or molecules that can damage cells as they seek to capture their missing electron—the murderer is a free radical whose crazed narrative of destruction triggers Nita's violent tale, which works: armed with what he takes to be incriminating information about her, the maniac takes the keys to her husband's car and drives away. Cancer, along with the unexpected death of her husband, has heightened Nita's awareness of the transience of human existence, but what rescues her are the powers of fiction.

Nita's fabricated story manages to neutralize the psychopath's true story. Whereas he had been deluded into believing in and acting on the paranoid fantasies in his head, she manipulates what she knows to be a false tale to save herself. Fiction understood as fiction is the antioxidant that defuses the free radicals of disease. Munro seems to subscribe to Anatole Broyard's view that "Stories are the antibodies against illness and pain." Not an escape from reality, fiction provides a temporary escape from death. True or false, the stories we tell about ourselves can become instrumental in shortening or extending our lives.

Lorrie Moore, an admirer of Alice Munro, is less sanguine about the relationship of narrative to cancer. The subtitle of Moore's most ambitious story about cancer gestures toward the problem of trying to use words to deal with disease. "People Like That Are the Only

People Here: Canonical Babbling in Peed Onk" is written in the third person and the present tense about the Mother and the Father and their Baby, who is diagnosed with a Wilms' tumor: "Is that apostrophe *s* or *s* apostrophe?" the Mother initially asks about the diagnosis, thinking, "Spelling can be important—perhaps even at a time like this, though she has never before been at a time like this, so there are barbarisms she could easily commit and not know."

The inanity of her response indicates that the shock of entering into the nightmare of pediatric oncology (Peed Onk) reduces the Mother and the Father to "canonical babbling": they time travel back to the sort of nonsensical vocalizing in gibberish that babies use before they acquire standardized language. Every conceivable narration of the catastrophe of a child's cancer—scientific, religious, artistic, personal—sounds ugly or funny or exploitative or feeble. And yet by documenting the failure of all this babble, Moore manages to convey the nightmare with extraordinary poignancy.

Hospital language frightens or alienates the Mother. When the Radiologist explains about the growth "You don't know exactly what it is until it's in the bucket," she sees "Swirls of bile and blood, mustard and maroon in a pail, the colors of an African flag or some exuberant salad bar: *in the bucket*—she imagines it all." Like the ugly phrase "Peed Onk," medical language can hardly be said to be appealing. Indeed, she thinks, "*Baby* and *Chemo* . . . they should never even appear in the same sentence together, let alone the same life." The Oncologist's phrase "a little light chemo" infuriates her: "*Eine Kleine* dactinomycin. I'd like to see Mozart write that one up for a big wad o' cash." The doctor-authored baby books at home never mention tumors, while the chirpy reassuring talk of hospital nurses and doctors—about the Baby having the best possible type of cancer—rings false to the Mother, who learns that the soothing pre-operative video about anesthesia hardly resembles the horror of watching the Baby being anesthetized.

When the Mother starts to pray "to some makeshift construction of holiness she has desperately, though not uncreatively, assembled in her mind," she finds herself bargaining with a "Higher Morality" in the likeness of "the manager at Marshall Field's sucking a Frango mint." This cosmic manager can only advise her that "the whole conception of 'the story,' of cause and effect, the whole idea that people have a clue as to how the world works is just a piece of laughable metaphysical colonialism perpetuated upon the wild country of time." About a baby getting cancer, she thinks with outrage "Who came up with *this* idea? What celestial abandon gave rise to *this*?" She believes that the other mothers of the "sweet, bald little angels" in the hospital want to say to God, "You can't have him! . . . You dirty old man! *Get out of here! Hands off!*" The Tiny Tim lounge they populate might have been less cramped if the celebrity's child had lived. The poky area bespeaks the celebrity's tangled feelings: "part gratitude, part generosity, part *fuck-you*."

While the Father continually instructs the Mother to take notes, because she is a creative writer and they will need the money, she demurs not only because "This isn't fiction" but also because "This is a nightmare of narrative slop. This cannot be designed." Even science fiction could not compete with, say, "leukemia, a tumor diabolically taking liquid form, better to swim about incognito in the blood. George Lucas, direct that!" In the waiting room during the Hickman implant and the nephrectomy and then in the recovery room, terror encases the Mother in mute horror so the narrator flounces on stage to ask derisively, "How can it be described?": "All that unsayable life! That's where the narrator comes in. The narrator comes in with her kisses and mimicry and tidying up. The narrator comes and makes a slow, fake song of the mouth's eager devastation." When the Baby's N-G tube fills with blood because the suction is too high, the attending physician looks to the Mother like a 15-year-old impersonating a doctor, making her believe that she's inside a musical comedy and "We've got Dr. 'Kiss Me Kate' here."

Less laughable than pathetic, the personal stories of the other parents who hope for the best or take one thing at a time strike the Mother as a bizarre response to the profound ethical dilemma that the pediatric oncology ward poses: namely, the suffering of the innocent. Her own stories of self-blame—she had cracked too many jokes about the "mind-wrecking chores, the same ones over and over again, like a novel by Mrs. Camus"—fail to alleviate her misery. The stoicism of the beleaguered parents astonishes but also upsets her. They "speak of other children's hospitals as if they were resorts," or they talk "not of the *possibility* of comas brought on by the chemo, but of the *number* of them."

Parents' stories about the miseries inflicted on children by treatment conclude with "strangely optimistic codas" tacked on. The Mother, who has become "addicted" to disaster tales, believes that the parents' accounts "leave Oprah in the dust." Although the Husband finds it comforting to find himself "in the same boat" with these "nice people with their brave stories," the Mother considers it a "nightmare boat." She leaps at the chance to leave, to have the Baby forgo chemotherapy and be monitored with ultrasound instead. Making her escape from Peed Onk, she never wants to see "any of these people again."

After a line break, the story ends with a punch line that feels to me like a punch in the gut:

THERE are the notes.
Now, where is the money?

Given the breakdown of almost all the interpolated narratives within Moore's story, the concluding words fume at the production of yet another (albeit drafty) account and at the impossibility of *not* constructing a story out of cancer trauma. Moreover, this ending accuses both writer and readers of what the literary critic Patricia Yaeger has called "consuming trauma." Fiction consumes us in absorbing attention, but we also consume it as a commodity: the author packages it for "a big wad o' cash," and we readers buy it for an Oprah moment.

For in response to the cancer of children, what else can any of us do except continue spewing out or gobbling up spurious beginnings and endings in stories that perpetuate the "laughable metaphysical colonialism perpetuated upon the wild country of time"? A rejoinder to cancer and its treatments, Lorrie Moore's story resembles the Tiny Tim lounge with its complicated message: "part gratitude, part generosity, part *fuck-you*." Those of us dismayed even by medical protocols that have saved or extended lives can value her courageous riposte, whether or not we agree with her.

In a nonfictional account of his 9-month-old daughter's catastrophic suffering from an atypical teratoid/rhabdoid tumor (A.T.R.T.), Aleksandar Hemon describes a trauma related to Moore's, but comes to a very different conclusion about his and his wife's isolation within the hospital, the new medical language they had to learn, the incomprehension of acquaintances, and the inanity of their platitudes as well as the unimaginable horror of emergency brain resections and chemo-induced fevers and seizures. After their baby's death, her "indelible absence" becomes "an organ in our bodies, whose sole function is a continuous secretion of sorrow."

Yet throughout the tragic ordeal, Hemon watches his older daughter, a 3-year-old, deal with it by making up stories about an imaginary brother through whom she can process her sister's illness. Although Hemon can cope with the baby's tribulations only by shutting down his imagination, his daughter Ella spins story after story. On the basis of her urgent need to unfurl these tales, Hemon concludes that "Narrative imagination—and therefore fiction—was a basic evolutionary tool of survival. We processed the world by telling stories, produced human knowledge through our engagement with imagined selves."

What about lyrical expressions that eschew the bogus cause and effect of plots, though they sometimes adopt imagined selves? Probably the least commercially profitable and most demanding artistic venture, poetry has always been uncannily at home with the sublime. Indisputably Ezra Pound was not thinking of poetry about cancer when he claimed that poetry is "news that STAYS news." William Carlos Williams turned my attention to Pound's famous maxim when I set out to write a news blog on contemporary poetry about cancer. "It is difficult / to get the news from poems," Williams wrote, "yet men die every day / for lack / of what is found there." I realized that the space limitations of a blog would make it impossible to represent the range of voices available in verse. But I also felt and still believe that this poetic tradition is only now emerging and that I do not have sufficient acumen to choose one text or author as more representative than any other.

Maureen McLane, in her book *My Poets*, discusses a poetic form—the cento—that solved my problem. It consists of snippets of verse composed by other writers. If assembled without attributions, it would be a plagiarist's dream. The genre speaks to me because I am a quilter who cuts out small bits of fabric to join to other small bits of fabric. Quilters call the process of sewing together different swatches of cotton "piecing." I set out to piece a cancer cento from the volumes of verse I had perused by stitching a line or two from one writer to a passage from another.

Readers who want to compose a cento of their own might start to keep a commonplace book or computer file: a collection of lines of verse that they encounter in their reading and that seem particularly meaningful. According to McLane, poets "make the chaos of inner feeling not only sentient but shareable." The chaos of feeling that surrounds disease differs for men and women subjected to quite different cancers. I therefore used verse by both men and women to convey a chaos of feeling that all of us can share.

Since there remains so much more reading and studying to do of creative texts that have received very little attention, it seems appropriate to conclude this preliminary meditation on cancer art with a slew of references sending you off to an abundance of writers who have struggled to articulate the awful fear and the fearful awe of cancer and its treatments. So with thanks to the authors who are footnoted below (with full references in the endnotes), here is an expanded version of the pieced poem I posted.

## A CANCER CENTO

My mouth opens and closes around the word cancer.[1]
Try saying *fear*. Now feel
Your tongue as it cleaves to the roof of your mouth.[2]
Once again I dress in white
paper and climb onto the table.[3]
Together we explore my inner landscape on the screen.
He plots a course and charts me frame by frame[4]—
like an X-ray
with here a mass and there a mass
and everywhere a mass.[5]
And then there's the blood tests. How many blood tests?
(Too many to count.)[6]
Negative = Positive, Positive = Negative = Bad.[7]


Even the surgeon who puts you to sleep
knows you will wake up robbed.[8]
What awaits you:
the leg bag, the IVs, the foreskin
looming like a skunk's tail,
and spasms like someone's driving a nail up your prick.[9]
Each wound speaks its own language.[10]

---

1  Joan Halperin, "Injunctions"
2  Alicia Suskin Ostriker, "The Mastectomy Poems"
3  Sandra Steingraber, "Outpatient"
4  Pat Borthwick, "Scan"
5  Christian Wiman, "Witness"
6  Lucia Perillo, "Needles"
7  Susan Deborah King, "Everywoman's Lexicon of Dread, with Commentary (Minimal)"
8  Pat Gray, "Cancer in the Breast"
9  Gustavo Pérez Firmat, "Post-Op"
10  Richard M. Berlin, "Wounds"

What is the splendor of one breast
on one woman?[11]

They've emptied your body of its enemies,
They're filling you with sterile juices.[12]
If Hell abides on earth this must be it:
This too-bright-lit-at-all-hours-of-the-day-
And-night recovery room, where nurses flit
In stroboscopic steps between the beds
All cheek by jowl that hold recoverers
Suspended in the grog of half-damped pain
And tubularities of light-blue light.[13]

I return across the darkened ward;
the grunts, coughs, and farts
sound as if I'm billeted on
an active volcano.[14]
The windows grow dark
and the grim snort
rasping from the next bed
never lets up, makes the night shudder.[15]
And poison, hung in sacks, began to drip. Poison
Doesn't last.[16]
Was it for this, *this*, become a *patient*, transformed to a
    shivering sack of blood to be spilled?

---

11  Lucille Clifton, "Consulting the Book of Changes: Radiation"
12  Sandra M. Gilbert, "For My Aunt in Memorial Hospital"
13  L. E. Sissman, "Homage to Clotho: A Hospital Suite"
14  Ifor Thomas, "Poleaxed"
15  Abba Kovnar, "The Windows Grow Dark"
16  Judith Hall, "Stamina"

And the dark night tracing of malevolent lymph tracks, fear
    scaling the ice-rungs of my spine?[17]

I need to see my tumour dead
A tumour which forgets to die
But plans to murder me instead.[18]
Swarm over him, my joy, my laughter, my Basic Life
Force! Let your bright sword-arm stream
Into that turgid hulk, worst
Of me growing.[19]
I don't know how to die yet. Let me live![20]

17   C. K. Williams, "Cancer"
18   Harold Pinter, "Cancer Cells"
19   James Dickey, "The Cancer Match"
20   Marilyn Hacker, "Cancer Winter"

Chapter 4

# My Blog

THE YEAR BEFORE I was supposed to die, I wanted to address the problems of cancer and its treatments with a larger group of readers. My oncologist had nailed every one of her earlier predictions. So, counting forward from the November 2008 diagnosis, I assumed the birth date on my gravestone would be linked to the death date 2013. November, which happens to be the month of my birthday, became an occasion for memento mori: an annual observance of my projected end. A statistical approximation, the prognosis tolled in my ears like a death sentence.

To my surprise, since 2012 I have been participating in a clinical trial and producing essays for the online *New York Times*. Every other Thursday at the beginning and now every month, I travel to the hospital for blood tests before receiving another batch of pills and posting a column in a series called "Living with Cancer." After more than two years, both events seem miraculous. The precious time the pills give me, the absorbing challenge the columns furnish: these are the unforeseen and joyful gifts that I do not want to attribute to cancer, because I begrudge its existence and bristle at any suggestion that such a pernicious disease can be considered a rewarding opportunity. They are gifts that I find fearful to record—I don't want to jinx them!—for there is no way of knowing how long they will last. It seems unlikely that I will remain in a chemically induced remission for the year of production it will take for you to be holding this book in your hands.

Back in 2012, my venture into journalism did not spring out of joy. While finishing a memoir about the treatments I received for ovarian cancer, I became obsessed with the need to raise consciousness about the lack of an early detection tool. More than 70 percent of ovarian cancers are discovered at later stages of the disease, which means that survival rates are poor. Indeed, of all cancers experienced by women, ovarian has the lowest five-year survival rate, because early symptoms can easily be misinterpreted or simply ignored. Bloating, constipation, satiety, fatigue: most middle-aged women are quite used to coping with and dismissing such seemingly trivial problems.

Misdiagnosis occurs when patients as well as doctors treat these symptoms as evidence of indigestion, menopause, irritable bowel syndrome, aging, or depression. Composing *Memoir of a Debulked Woman* enabled me to rant at length about the need to develop better detection tools and also about the miserable treatments to which women with ovarian cancer are subjected. But book buyers remain a small percentage of the public. How could I reach more people? I wanted to write differently—not scholarly tomes but easily accessible and, if possible, widely circulated essays.

I therefore composed one short journalistic piece and searched the Web for ideas about where to send it. The search depressed me. I treasure literary reviews and journals, but their readership tends to be small and mostly academic. When I perused popular women's magazines, the "we-can-beat-cancer" brass band put me off. Too many articles composed by self-defined role models, cheerleaders, and advice givers perpetuate the idea that if patients cultivate a "good attitude" and a "fighting spirit," they can cure themselves and become "cancer free." My 3,000-word essay—I have no idea how I came to believe that this was an appropriate length—included disturbing material about the suffering and physical dysfunctions caused by cancer treatments.

Now, I realize that I was trapped in a repetition compulsion, trying to cram into that essay all the grotesque events I had recounted in the memoir. At the start of July 2012, though, I sent it with an email to Charles McGrath at the *New York Times*, in the hope that he would remember assigning me a few book reviews in the 1980s. He put me in touch with an editor at the *New York Times Magazine* who was kind enough to offer editorial suggestions; but the piece was, of course, unsuitable for her purposes.

Meanwhile, I was reading with admiration Suleika Jaouad's online blog in the electronic *Times*. The candid, smart posts in her series "Life, Interrupted" dealt with Suleika's leukemia treatments and taught me that my macabre condensation of the memoir would be too dreary for any newspaper. I therefore drafted a short piece protesting upbeat cancer survivor rhetoric that makes people with chronic or terminal disease feel like losers.

On August 7, 2012, I sent off "On Not Being a Cancer Survivor" to the health editor at the *Times* and heard back immediately from Tara Parker-Pope, the editor of the online Well section. She thought it could be turned into two essays. After some quick revision, the next week I was in the weird position of waiting to hear if Tara Parker-Pope liked the pieces and if blood work and a CT scan would make me eligible for a Phase I clinical trial of a promising experimental drug. The essays were accepted just as I was accepted into the trial. The confluence of the two events contributed to my euphoria.

From conversations in my cancer support group, which had started up a month earlier, I had some ideas about additional submissions. After I sent Tara Parker-Pope a few more essays, she emailed to ask if I would be interested in posting regularly. Suleika Jaouad, it turned out, needed time off during her treatments, and we could take turns. Suleika had morphed from a teacher into a colleague or teammate. I remember exactly where I was when I received this proposal on my iPhone. My husband Don and I were on the highway, driving back from the Simon Cancer Center in Indianapolis to Bloomington, and I was so exalted that we stopped at, yes, a Wendy's to celebrate.

The greatest thrill came from the prospect of my words appearing in the electronic edition of a newspaper I had venerated since a child. It was Tara Parker-Pope's idea to call the series "Living with Cancer." Despite the composition quandaries that ensued, I am deeply indebted to her for coming up with such a hospitable venue, and also for editorial support that has sustained me. Though I have worked with excellent editors on numerous books, she has been the most brilliant at helping me pitch my work to a specific audience.

Over the mounting months and now years, the pleasures and the problems I encountered while writing the column have convinced me that the Internet offers prodigious resources for patient advocacy, but it also circumscribes and compromises personal expression. The blog has made me aware, as no other sort of writing has, of the sometimes deleterious influence of readers' expectations on writers. My foray into journalism has taught me about the powers and the limitations of blogging and also about my own failings.

Yet despite my failures, I remain convinced that the small and humble form of the blog can be mined by people with various experiences of disease in creative and deeply satisfying ways. So after probably too much grousing and chest-beating, in this chapter I do eventually get around to offering some ideas on how prospective bloggers might use generative but simple formats to structure and enrich their essays.

To begin with, the column was exhilarating because it felt like the opposite of scholarly writing. Whereas my academic essays often took months, if not years, to compose, a blog could be drafted in a few days. Academic articles often include thirty pages of dense and heavily footnoted prose, but the blog was supposed to be about three double-spaced pages, or about 850 words. A tidy blog seemed preferable to a baggy monster because I could capture one ephemeral response to cancer treatments without making a big deal about its universality or its staying power.

Given the contradictory and complicated series of reactions I and many others undergo during treatment, I was grateful that the modesty of the form impeded the sorts of generalizations that can depress cancer patients. Also, because chronic cancer patients like me do not know how long we will be able to keep cancer at bay, the quick tempo of blog publishing felt more suitable to my needs than the stately pace of print publishing.

While academic essays take months to be accepted, having to pass first through outside readers and editorial boards, judgment on the blog posting (attached to an email) is immediate. I rarely got paid for writing a scholarly essay, but with every blog I logged into an electronic freelance account to get paid, which made me feel like a professional. (Of course if I had gone into writing to pay the bills, I would have hanged myself years ago.) Although I often had to wait months for responses to my criticism in print, on the blog readers posted comments immediately. Even the rejection of an early essay motivated me to continue posting. It contained an allusion to the tragic murder of children in a Sandy Hook elementary school. When Tara Parker-Pope explained her refusal to include any reference to that horrific occurrence in the Well section, I felt freed in subsequent posts to ignore the most gruesome current events so as to focus exclusively on the issues of cancer.

At the start, the thrills and chills of journalism, especially for an academic, had everything to do with daredevil timing. Often the editing occurred on a Thursday morning while I was traveling to the Indianapolis hospital or was inside it. The iPhone would bing and there would be the changes proposed by TPP, as my family started to call her. Never expert on the tiny keyboard, I would laboriously respond point by point to each altered word, each phrase queried, each concluding paragraph slashed. Since the piece would be posted that afternoon, I had to react immediately, whether I was on the highway or in a cubicle waiting to see my oncologist. Don always drove and advised me, but the pace was unnerving. I soon began to send my essays to TPP on Wednesdays in the hope that the back-and-forth negotiating over revisions could begin before I left for the hospital.

As I eased into this freelance job, it made sense to draft essays whenever ideas came to me. In the past I had avoided deadlines; I did not want to be stressed over not having material ready. OK, that's not the whole story. Maybe because my background on both maternal and paternal sides is German Jewish, I always arrive fifteen minutes early for a class or lecture and always had fellowship applications ready weeks before they were due. As a writer, I am an inveterate reviser. So in the fall of 2012 I set to work every day sketching ideas for future columns or fiddling with drafted versions. Pretty soon I had a backlog of essays that I could rework over and over again. The idea was to make them so tightly constructed that TPP could only tinker.

To produce nonacademic prose, I worked continuously on shorter paragraphs, simpler word choices, less convoluted sentence patterns, and also on the ordering of the essays, which I listed in a document called "Column Order." I knew that readers of an online newspaper would probably not keep track of what I had posted two weeks or a month ago, but I needed to think about the logic of the sequence. Sometimes the order was determined by what historians would call material conditions. For example, if an article on yoga appeared in the Well section that week, I would postpone my essay on yoga for cancer patients so it would not look repetitive. Or if one of my essays included new information on the efficacy of the drug in my trial or the arrival of a grandchild, it moved up on the list so the post would quickly reflect a change in my life.

Even though some of the essays existed on my computer months before I sent them, I wanted readers to have up-to-date knowledge of my medical condition and family situation. At other times, the logic pertained to an upcoming holiday or to tone—seeking to avoid a succession of depressing posts, for example. I had set out to counter the usual "we-can-beat-cancer" hype that whitewashes the misery of the disease and its treatments, but I also did not want to turn off readers with nothing but doom and gloom.

The illustration that TPP found for each blog often illuminated my words. In the case of *The SCAR Project*, her decision to reproduce several of David Jay's extraordinary photographs of breast cancer patients lent power to the column. That blogs can so easily include graphics or links to graphics turned my attention to other visual artists who could not have been easily discussed in a journal or book format, given the expense of color reproductions. At times, however, the illustrations unnerved me, as did the impossibility of footnoting thinkers to whom I was indebted, the deletion of swear words even in quotations, the retitling of my essays, and (admittedly) some of those slashed paragraphs. The biggest struggles, though, arose not from editorial decisions but within me, and they involved self-editing—or perhaps it would be better to call it self-censorship.

I alluded to the issue of self-editing or self-censorship earlier when I mentioned not wanting to post a succession of unrelenting doom-and-gloom columns. From comments about my memoir that appeared on Amazon.com, I knew that my pessimism about what I took to be my incurable state upset readers desperately wanting to sustain hope about their own or a relative's diagnosis. In the "Living with Cancer" series, I had to be true to my sense of my condition without presuming that my skepticism about cancer cures should be bottled and sold. Unlike free writing, writing online involves not only self-expression but also an awareness of readers—of their situations, needs, and wants. Self-editing or self-censorship took place for a variety of reasons and in positive as well as negative ways, all related to the very public nature of posting very personal essays in a medium with such wide reach.

Starting with positive self-editing enables me to acknowledge the powerful influence and input of the members of my cancer support group. Every two weeks this group meets for lunch to discuss the various problems and challenges each of us faces with a gynecological cancer. I always attend with a pad and a pen, because the discussions often find their way into columns. When we began, I had warned the six others that I was a writer, but promised that I would be circumspect in representing their issues in print so that their privacy would be preserved. From this group of courageous women, I have learned how differently people react to the decision making, symptoms, side effects, and surveillance inevitably confronting cancer patients during ongoing treatment.

All of the women in the group are younger than I and more committed to trying complementary approaches in addition to standard medical care. They get massages, engage acupuncturists, work out with trainers, read up on mistletoe injections, gather turkey tail mushrooms, brew teas, try Chinese herb extracts, and purchase supplements. My friends engage in these pursuits knowing they are not curative, but hoping they might produce some physiological or psychological benefit. Who can argue with that? Who would want to argue with that? Although skeptical about alternative approaches, I allowed myself to sample at least some of them when I pretended to put myself in a role hilariously at odds with my actual situation: that of investigative reporter.

After all, I told myself, complementary therapies might be of use to readers of the blog, and they would be an interesting way to circumvent what I feared would become my knee-jerk nay-saying. Little did I know that I would stick with the yoga class for cancer patients that I attended in order to write a column. Never could I have suspected that I would sign up for a workshop called "Look Good, Feel Better" and then, months later, actually use some of the makeup. Only because a member of the support group had gotten a wig did I decide to try one, wear it regularly, and write several columns about so-called cranial prostheses. The avenues suggested by the support group helped me keep cancer in the news, even though for weeks and months living with cancer can be just as stunningly banal as living without cancer.

A more negative source of self-editing or self-censorship I will encapsulate in the phrase "Drink the carrot juice." To understand it, you need to factor in the effect of readers' responses—both their nature and their number. In the Well section, next to the title of every column a number appears to indicate how many responses have been posted. Chalk it up to my competitive spirit, but unfortunately this number quickly became an obsession. A paragraph or two on leaving toe fungus untreated or on nightly urination would receive hundreds of responses, whereas what I considered my finely strung pearls of wisdom would get a pitiful fraction of that total.

I had vowed never to respond to the responders, but I read them avidly and the most heartfelt made me weep. Most reader comments were and are smart and generous. But like student evaluations at the end of the semester, the ones that stay with me are the uncongenial comments, and at times they inhibited the truthfulness that personal writing entails. Some version of "Drink the carrot juice" popped up recurrently, whether I was writing about insomnia or about the insertion of a port.

Well-meaning readers posted notes with website links on the curative power of five cups of carrot juice daily and also promised me that patients should be confident that they can always be the person they want to be. Others warned against the evils of standard medical care or of sleeping pills or talcum powder, and the importance of—you name it—supplements, vitamins, a Mexican healer, a particular brand of shoes, medicinal cannabis, and, very often, carrots. Especially after a disturbing column on, say, the numb extremities caused by chemotherapy, people provided pragmatic solutions. I appreciated their suggestions, but sensed that they expected me to follow suit, to produce advice columns with practical instructions. However, I was interested in exploring the hopes, fears, and uncertainties of patients. I had neither the temperament nor the expertise to dole out advice (except, as I have in these pages, about writing and reading).

A related trigger of self-censorship—let's call it "Smile, you have cancer!"—probably originates out of the understandable desire of many readers for inspirational words. Curiously, those who want cancer patients to be merry tend to be very angry people indeed. Since upsetting essays generated meaner reader responses, I found myself muting or glossing over some of the more grotesque effects of treatment. Many bloggers must deal with the insults of "trolls" (responders—often anonymous or pseudonymous—who deliberately provoke fights), though surely there are fewer of them in the Well section than on political blogs. On- and off-site, however, I received some disturbing responses.

One arrived an hour after I posted a blog about cleaning out my university office and home closets so as to relinquish my old identities and make space for new ones, especially for the sort of joy I experience (described at the end of the column) over the birth of a grandson. Since I considered this to be a realistic assessment of losses followed by a happy gain, I was not prepared for an email sent to the *Times'* editorial staff and copied to me:

Healthy people declutter.
Feng Shui is a design choice.
This maudlin self-indulgent self-pitying cloying writing is unbe-

coming to a former intelligent writer, and discouraging to
other cancer patients.
No one is interested in never-ending whining and her display of
dirty laundry
Please can this column

Call me thin-skinned, but this letter turned me into a maudlin, self-indulgent, and self-pitying whiner. (Not cloying, though,
I tried to reassure myself.) It was neither better nor worse than a
subsequent email forwarding the judgment of another reader who
found everything I wrote "dark and nasty."

Both "Drink the carrot juice" and "Smile, you have cancer!"
tempted me to convey what patients are supposed to feel, not what
I in fact did feel. Should I tidy up my thoughts to conform to
the expectations of Well readers, many of whom have pledged allegiance to healthy lifestyles—diet, exercise, keeping up to date on
medically approved methods of monitoring the body? In a con-
temptible need to obtain and keep the attention of readers, would
I repress or lie about my sometimes unhealthy habits and perverse
mind-sets?

An example may illustrate how at times I did collude in producing
just the sort of sunny advice-giving type of cancer writing that I had set
out to resist. In "Hospital City," I sketched the various ways in which
hospitals intensify the indignities and terrors of patients. One person
complained about my whining (yup, there's that word again) and wondered if the author thought she was the first person who ever had cancer. The essay gave her the idea, she added, that the author felt entitled
not to suffer these indignities and terrors. Actually, I do believe we are
entitled to better environments than the ones we find in contemporary
hospitals, big and small. (Just think of hospital food!)

Although I had begun the blog with the conviction that honesty about the harsh realities of treatment was what I could add to conversations about cancer, after I read that comment about my whiny entitlement I set out to write a very pragmatic column listing specific remedies for the depression that chemotherapy often brings in its wake. I knew that many patients succumb to depression and that at times I had found nothing able to resist it; however, the pressure of readers' expectations was simply too great. People want cancer patients to be optimistic and resourceful about what they must endure. When I reread that column, it still seems alien to my fundamentally glum sense that respites are hard to come by.

In fact, it teeters perilously close to a parody I produced to mock the sort of bubbly self-help magazine articles found in doctors' waiting rooms. Here is a copy of that lampoon, which I never submitted since my brilliant first editor, my husband, did not think readers would get the joke unless I opened with the explanation that it was a satire (which would have ruined it for me).

## COOK ON CHEMO!

Working step by step, you can cook on chemo! Marshal your forces and put on a happy face! What better way to begin than Jewish penicillin: aka Chicken Noodle Soup? You just have to plan—one week ahead of time. So here's the countdown.

Day 1—Set the table for as many as it seats. The table set for a big occasion means you cannot sit down and eat. That's what we call a mitzvah (a blessing), the first of many that come from cooking on chemo.

Day 2—Make a grocery list while you wait for the surgeon to answer your emailed questions: one chicken, celery, carrots, two boxes of chicken stock (or a jar of bouillon cubes), a bag of noodles, and a few cans of Campbell's chicken soup. It is *always* cheery to make a to-do list! You will check it off later, but now it's time to go get that blood transfusion.

Day 3—Grab your wig or hat, we're off to the supermarket. The fresh air and exercise will do you no end of good! Here's a second mitzvah (blessing)—no need to buy organic: The damage is already done! Remember, there is a chair near the checkout line and the bathroom is behind the meat department. Be sure to cover your drainage bulbs, external catheters, or trach. Being considerate of others is a mitzvah (a blessing)!

Day 4—During infusion, check off the items on your grocery list and you will have accomplished something *already*! Still, you need to meditate and visualize like crazy because tomorrow is huge. Reschedule the endoscopy-and-colonoscopy combo for the following week. Ditto the cystogram. Insurance forms can wait.

Day 5—Deal with your gag reflex while taking the chicken out of its packaging by singing "These Are a Few of My Favorite Things." Plunk it in a big pot and put the pot on the burner before pouring in the water cup by cup: Otherwise it will be too heavy to lift! To avoid passing out, lean against the counter to scrape a carrot and skin an onion. After popping them in the pot, phone the surgeon's receptionist with a reminder about your questions (so as not to pass out).

When you hear the water boiling, go back to the stove. Hold your nose with one hand and with the other skim off the gunk on the top. (If you cannot handle a utensil, skip this step.) Lower the flame before you pass out as the soup simmers for a few hours.

No biggie if you forgot the soup! Should that happen, salvage what chicken you can and throw out the rest. You have boxes of stock (or a jar of cubes) at hand. All's well that ends well: Skip to Day 7.

If you remembered the soup, WOW!! KUDOS!! You need to take the chicken off the bone and throw out the skin, but tomorrow is another day so put it on a trivet. Prayer is a fabulous mitzvah (blessing): Pray that the chicken doesn't go rancid overnight.

Day 6—You help others when you let them help you! After reheating the pot, ask a neighbor to pour its contents through a colander into a container, toss the veggies, and place the chicken in front of your chair with a garbage bag by your feet. Look to see that steam is not rising from the chicken: Even though you can't feel your fingers, you can still burn them! Do yoga breathing while removing chicken and tossing bones and gristle. Put some of the chicken back into the broth and refrigerate. Give the rest to your neighbor for chicken salad—giving to others is a big mitzvah (blessing)!

Day 7—Congratulations! You made it from scratch. Oops—hope that didn't trigger your rashes! After skimming off the fat on top of the stock, pour it into a pot. If mouth sores permit, add salt and pepper. Then heat to a simmer (or heat the boxes or the cubes in water). Add noodles and set a timer for ten minutes: A timer is the chemo-cook's best friend!

Don't have a timer or do have hearing loss and the broth evaporated? No problemo! Simply toss the burnt noodles or if they
are stuck to the pot, toss the pot. You've got your Campbell's
and you know what to do: Go to bed.

Can't sleep? Concerned about weight loss? Get take out!
Another tip: Call it take in.

Here's a final mitzvah (blessing)—you can dream about next
month's column: Icy Hockey on Chemo!

P.S. Write in with other suggestions for this exciting series!

To alleviate my obsession with blog responses, I kept a gift from one
of my daughters on the end table next to the blue couch. She had
taped onto a yellow piece of construction paper a *New Yorker* cartoon
by Ward Sutton. In it, a psychiatrist advises a patient on the couch,
"Let's try focussing on your posts that *do* receive comments." Laugh-
ing at myself helped, but not enough. At the risk of revealing my
depraved nature, I confess that I asked a number of friends to post
retorts to the crueler responses to my essays. Most of them, however,
found the idea absurd.

Still, I remained obsessed. Suleika Jaouad always received
many more posted responses than I did, especially if she discussed
her puppy. (I included that last bit to show you how odious I had
become.) Unbeknownst to her, I fell into a ridiculous and doomed
rivalry—hard to admit, because this admirable young woman
wrote heroically about her bone marrow transplant. At one point, I
became so insufferable to myself that I offered to quit. Only assur-
ances from TPP that she would never judge the quality of an essay

by the number of posted responses saved me from throwing in the towel.

Since I was supposed to be writing personal essays, another kind of censorship—let's call this one "I may have cancer, but I'm no expert"—surfaced when I became obsessed with the story of a Texas woman dealing with ovarian cancer. After multiple surgeries, sessions of chemotherapy, radiation, and a stem cell transplant, Andrea Sloan went on a mission to change the byzantine, hard-to-negotiate system by which very sick patients petition for what is called compassionate use: permission to obtain an unapproved, experimental drug when no others work. Her effort to get a medication being offered in clinical trials (for which she was ineligible) had galvanized many people on the Internet.

Given Andrea Sloan's conviction that only this drug could save her, I sympathized with her plight. Yet I worried about the drafted column because I know so little about the regulations of the FDA. So I asked my oncologist to check out what I had written. When she argued that compassionate use in this case could impede ongoing research without prolonging Andrea Sloan's life, I decided that I did not have the authority to serve as her advocate. I first rewrote the column to record the limits of my understanding, and then ditched it. I had and have no wish to become a faux journalist or ersatz science reporter.

The most powerful sort of self-censorship at work in blog writing resembles the self-policing that must plague anyone engaged in writing a memoir or autobiography and aware of the ethics of self-revelation. My story is never *just* my story: it involves family, friends, colleagues, physicians, nurses, and acquaintances. And of course their privacy must be respected. In this regard, Suleika—a stunning brunette—became not my teacher, teammate, or rival but a foil: her character stood in marked contrast to mine. She included pictures and videos of herself, sometimes with her brother or mother, sometimes with a boyfriend, sometimes with a fellow cancer patient or a nurse, and clearly with their consent. Most of the people in my circle regarded that sort of exposure with horror. Nor did I want to display pictures of myself, given the grotesque toll of treatment.

Even my experiences as a cancer patient had to be censored if they would embarrass me or distress my caregivers. In my memoir I wrote about various hospital mishaps and mistakes, naming the doctors who had hurt rather than helped me. But I worried about posting *Times* columns in which I discussed incompetent or harried nurses or botched surgeries. It was clear to me that quite a few people on the staff at the hospital in which I receive care were reading my blogs, and I certainly did not want to hurt any individual's feelings. Also, I feared retribution.

If I sullied the reputation of the hospital, which was in the process of extending my life, might retaliation come by way of punitive or (just as unnerving) unfriendly caretaking? I could cope with that fear by attributing it to paranoia and also by framing my criticisms in the context of the lifesaving work the hospital performs not only for me but for many others. Still, another topic remained more intransigent. I dwell on it here because many patients with cancer face taboos that make them fearful that what they need to discuss may be too gross or too frightful for other people to read.

Let's zoom in to focus on a subject that Virginia Woolf once called the difficulty of telling the truth about the body and that became for me the difficulty of writing truthfully about complicated reactions to the body in treatment. One of the requisites of the genre of the blog, after all, is pacing: the first sentences must set up a proposition or recount an incident that is demonstrated or clarified in the 850 words that follow. There is no room for a succession of passionate yet conflicting attitudes, because only one mood, or at the most two, can be caught in three typed pages. Yet patients often cycle through multiple emotional loops as they endure and then live through major medical upheavals.

My feelings about the ileostomy that I had undergone in February 2009—which brought a segment of the small intestine through the abdominal wall to form a stoma—lurched over a number of years from deep revulsion and outrage to disgust, shame, and then to half-hearted resignation. It seemed wrong to gloss over the revulsion, outrage, disgust, and shame so as to settle on the resignation or to leap to what most people would probably prefer to read about, an acceptance that I (alas) have never fully achieved. Writing about embarrassing aspects of my body in a broadly distributed medium freaked me out. Did I really want my colleagues all around the country to know about my daily problems with poop?

Although I had written about the ileostomy in my memoir, I was worried that a blog on that topic would embarrass me and upset my kids. A few pages about having to wear a bag that collects excrement are one thing in a book, but quite another in the most-read online newspaper in America. In the book, I could hint at my hope that the operation might be reversed, but now I knew it wouldn't be. I had discovered the blog of an earlier *Times* columnist, Dana Jennings, who discussed his permanent ileostomy but always in the context of his gratitude: it saved him from suffering. He did not share my sense of loathing at the nauseating mess of perpetually dealing with shit. At the beginning of my first draft of "Stoma Stigma," I tried to tell the truth about my reticence. Here are the opening paragraphs:

## STOMA STIGMA

Most of you don't know us and we don't know each other. Silenced by modesty or embarrassment, only a few have expressed their alienation from or acceptance of an operation that saved our lives. Can I evolve from estrangement to acquiescence?

If you have ever used a blow dryer on your stomach, if you fear fouling the bed, if you leave the house with a kit containing wipes, a plastic pouch, a tube of paste, and a flange, you are probably one of the 500,000 Americans with a temporary or permanent colostomy, ileostomy, or urostomy. We are called osto*mates*, though some of us feel like singular anomalies. Physicians assure ostomates that we can travel, engage in sex and sports, wear and eat what we want. What well-meaning advisors rarely discuss is the sense of shame that can plague recovery after such surgery.

After explaining that the word "stoma" means mouth and what an ileostomy entails and who undergoes the operation for what sorts of conditions, I ended "Stoma Stigma" by discussing first an artist who uses her art to deal with her outrage at having to live with an ostomy and then a more accepting celebrity memoirist. Here is that conclusion:

One visual artist, Carol Chase Bjerke, has produced a series of installations protesting "a crude and outdated procedure that continues to serve as standard treatment for a variety of gastrointestinal diseases." To dramatize the compulsion to conceal such an indignity, "Intimate Apparel" puts on display the usually hidden ostomy pouch as if it were a delicate piece of lingerie.

Also photographed in her book *Hidden Agenda*, "Misfortune Cookies" consists of 150 polymer clay stomas, each (about 1¼ inch by 1¼ inch by 1¾ inch) placed next to the others in rows and each spouting a narrow strip of paper from its central opening. On the paper strips journal entries are translated into the second person of fortune cookies.

The misfortunes emitted from these dark red mouths bespeak anger, frustration, nausea, and impotence:

"You will be saved and betrayed."
"You have a wound that will not heal."
"You will be sick to DEATH of handling your own excrement."
"You will want to eliminate the process of elimination."
"You will have a secret."

Visited with unjust deserts, Bjerke hopes that alternative methods of treatment will be devised so that a mortifying protocol can become obsolete.

The actress Barbara Barrie initially shared this sense of mortification at "my intestines blatantly exposed—glistening with moisture and actual feces." After cancer of the rectum and a herniated stoma, she wrote, "I was subhuman, a leper, something to be thrown out." Yet eventually in her memoir *Second Act*, she exults that her body "began to function in its own new way." Indeed, as she continues to perform on stage she has "become very fond of this colostomy . . . because it's freeing, it's my gate to health."

Like Bjerke and Barrie, I endorse the theme of last October's World Ostomy Day: "Let's Be Heard." I wasn't ready to celebrate then, but who knows about 2013? In the interim, expressing the inexpressible—in our various ways—may serve as one means of making that agenda visible.

. . . . . . . . . . . . . . . . . . . . . . . . . . . . . . . . . . . . . . . . . . . . . . . . . . . . . . . . . . . . . . . . . . . . . . .

This essay stayed on my computer and kept on moving down the "Column Order" list. I could not imagine TPP reproducing the brilliant but explicit artwork of Carol Chase Bjerke, and I feared censorious comments from readers living happily ever after with ostomies. Worse, might my words depress or frighten people who have to undergo this sort of surgery? Because I do not deal well with repression, I wrote a long essay titled "Stumped" that I never sent out for publication but that directly addressed the source of my disgust.

In it, I go on and on about how "it is impossible to be naked— except briefly in the shower where I focus my eyes downward and see what should be inside sticking out. The stoma looks like a sort of degraded or castrated penis, the tip of an udder, or an out-of-place nipple. Although I fast for at least sixteen hours before a shower, I keep watch on the stoma in case of leaks so I can clean up the tub before my husband notices droppings. . . . Then anxiety arises about reddening skin around the stoma from the paste under the flange: what if the skin should break down? I shudder considering the total catastrophe that would ensue, if I could not make the pouch stick to my body."

I also describe mishaps: "accidents are the worst, plunging me into gloom. About once a month, a flange unhinges from my belly, thereby unhinging me into panicky curses: 'Shit!' or 'crap!' unimaginatively trips off my tongue. Sobs must be stifled so I can immediately clean myself up." Sometimes exactly what we cannot express to family and friends needs to be put down in words.

But if the ostomy involved such distress, why was I deeming the subject unacceptable for the *Times*? I felt particularly guilty about my self-censorship when a friend in my support group needed help. Avastan—an experimental drug being tested on women with ovarian cancer—caused a bowel perforation and she had to undergo an ileostomy. Seeing how few resources were at her disposal, I rewrote "Stoma Stigma" and determined to submit it; however, I diluted my own disgust so as not to alienate readers. Here is that revised blog:

## STOMA STIGMA

Over the past year and a half, I have tried to be candid in this column, but one matter seemed inexpressible: an operation that saved my life so mortified me that I drafted many essays without being able to post any of them. Then a member of my cancer support group underwent the same surgery and asked me for help.

At my first visit to her house, Marie said, "I have dealt with ovarian cancer for five years, but I have never been so frustrated, so close to an emotional breakdown, as with this thing. What if it happens in a public place? It takes half an hour to clean myself up. And then there's the laundry."

What Marie meant by "this thing" is a stoma, the bit of small intestine pulled out of the body during an ileostomy and then stitched onto the stomach. From the Greek word meaning "mouth," the stoma—a dark red protuberance, an inch in diameter, jutting out on one side below the waist—emits excrement from a small hole at its center. What Marie meant by "if it happens" is an accident when the appliance malfunctions and waste oozes out of the pouch onto her body and clothes. I understood how fraught she felt because I periodically contend with the same dread and mess.

After various types of ostomy surgery, a number of people react with relief, rather than revulsion, because the stoma alleviates agonies caused by a range of maladies: injuries, ulcerative colitis, Crohn's disease, colorectal or bladder cancers. For those suffering with recurrent diarrhea, constipation, incontinence, or acute abdominal pains, the surgical construction of a bypass bestows a modicum of respite and control. This sort of operation indisputably rescues patients from torment and even from death.

To underscore how valiantly many children, teenagers, and adults rise to the challenge of dealing with a stoma, I want to contrast them to Marie and me. We had never suffered chronic intestinal pain and therefore experienced more revulsion than relief. Cancer treatment necessitated our ileostomies: Marie acquired her stoma after an experimental drug produced a fistula; I got mine after a botched surgery triggered a series of infections.

The injury to physiological integrity and autonomy can be shocking. Coping with a leaky body and with constant upkeep is demoralizing. Like me, Marie feels humiliated by the filth with which she has to contend. She worries that under some circumstances she may have neither the privacy nor the dexterity to deal with all the equipment—a pouching system, tubes of paste, skin barriers, adhesive removers, wipes—and therefore she dreads a constricted existence.

Over 500,000 Americans survive with temporary or permanent colostomies, ileostomies, and urostomies, yet there are very few personal accounts: Eve Ensler's recent memoir *In the Body of the World* is the exception that proves the rule. Surgeons assure us that we can travel, engage in sex and sports, wear and eat what we want. What well-meaning advisors rarely discuss is the sense of shame that can plague recovery. The silence around the subject would stun me, except that I have also been tempted to sustain it.

Only with the help of ostomy nurses could I master the rigorous maintenance a stoma requires. I urged Marie to avail herself of these angelic assistants and of another aid that I only recently discovered on the Internet.

Online chat venues dedicated to every type of cancer are beneficial, but on a taboo subject they can be a real boon. Web-based ostomy support groups and discussion boards contain posts about very specific problems that are then addressed by other patients who provide detailed suggestions on what to do about leaks, on how to find comfortable or camouflaging clothing, on strategies to avoid skin breakdown, on how to time the changing of bags, on whether mushrooms, corn, cauliflower, or nuts should be avoided.

Online "ostomates" comfort each other and encourage themselves to record the unspeakable—always with compassion, sometimes with levity. Maybe because the stoma requires round-the-clock care, like a newborn, quite a few people name their stomas: sometimes simply Fred or Bruce; sometimes, given its color, Rosy or Scarlet; sometimes, quite understandably, Chaos, Sir Poops, Droopy, or Stumpy. "A bag is better than a box," they joke among themselves.

In the meantime, Marie has gained confidence with a new functioning apparatus. And gritty conversations with her and on websites have emboldened me to breach the silence surrounding stoma stigma. Maybe it's time to broaden the discussion.

Yet I continue to dream of the day when children, teenagers, and adults with alimentary ailments can be freed without being fouled. Though my shame shames me, for some of us this subject remains more fraught than any other aspect of living with cancer.

. . . . . . . . . . . . . . . . . . . . . . . . . . . . . . . . . . . . . . . . . . . . . . . . . . . . . . . . .

Even in this modulated fashion, letting the world know about my abjection frightened me, though I felt and still feel strongly that the struggles of people dealing with interminable and degrading upkeep should be made known. The second version of "Stoma Stigma" also never got posted. Ah, the sleazy passive voice creeps in! Let me rephrase: I simply lacked the courage to submit this essay to TPP. On the Internet, I failed to solve the problem of writing truthfully about my body.

The playwright Eve Ensler's reaction to her stoma—"this little fleshy nipple made me feel suddenly maternal"—had astonished me. She associates its "birth announcement" with "The End of My Invincibility" and celebrates "how this exposure, this shit-filled nipple of my vulnerability, was the pathway to mercy." Surely this is a more psychologically healthy and ethically responsible reaction than mine. Later, on an online mail list sent to me daily called Team Inspire, I read posts from participants in the ostomy group: "How to help 6-year-old after ileostomy reversal?"

and "Does anyone have 2 bags to contend with?" I became further shamed by my shame.

Why can I publish what I cannot post? Perhaps I will be dying or dead by the time this book is printed, but in any case I will not have to deal with the instantaneous responses of readers. And perhaps an account of my failures will pave the way for the successes of future writers. Or maybe tomorrow or the next day I will find a way to address this vexed problem—without self-pity or embarrassment and without harming those who must also cope with it. This hope springs from the genuine delight I took in a novel I just read, Bernardine Bishop's *Unexpected Lessons in Love*, about a therapist with anal cancer and a writer with bowel cancer, both with colostomies.

Hello—delight? Yes, for as these two friends deal with their anxieties about stomas and cancer, all the amazing stuff and staffs of life—adopted babies and sexual desires and voluntarily chosen family ties—take over. Even in the face of a recurrence, the novelist character is "stunned and impressed that the writing urge should be strong enough to counteract the panic urge": "But it was. And the fact that it was, was in itself emboldening." Because Bishop found a way to write truthfully and poignantly about characters with ostomies, I am convinced that "the writing urge" will impel future cancer patients to do what I failed to do—to overcome taboos and, without grossing out or frightening readers, compose essays about what has been unspeakable.

Often addressing personal matters, the blog has been a form especially suitable for cancer patients. The concentration blogging demands and the communication it affords can help anyone who wants to experiment with this new and malleable genre. If you plug "how to blog" into your search engine, a number of websites will explain the mechanisms of setting up a site. Any one of the prompts offered in the first chapter of this book might serve as a springboard for a blog. Actually, a single prompt—like "Untie the strands of a domestic or work-related knot created by treatment" or "Yesterday or today, I found myself puzzled or inspired by . . ."—could generate a series of short essays. Similarly, any one of the memoirs discussed in the second chapter and any one of the narratives and images discussed in the third chapter could stimulate responses that take the form of a blog.

I have found it helpful to approach such topics by trying standard formats that have been mined by generations of expository writers. Flexible templates, they should be used only as long as they help you arrange your sentences and paragraphs; if and when they become a hindrance, they should be jettisoned in favor of the organization that is emerging through the writing process. Here is a list of suggested strategies that you can use to structure your response to a prompt or to any subject upon which you want to deliberate in a short essay.

> Pose a cancer-related problem and propose a solution: set out a question you faced, exploring its facets, and then explain how you have answered it or moved away from it.

> Argue for a specific improvement in cancer care, being sure to address the objections that might be raised against it.

> Describe a medical environment and conclude with what it signifies to you: stick to a sarcastic, lyrical, or objective style and then consider switching the tone in your final remarks.

Discuss a decision turnabout: begin with your conviction about a particular set of treatment paths and then explain why you have changed your mind, or why you don't understand why you changed your mind and what that tells you about yourself or your situation.

Tell a story about a domestic or social event: narrate the specific incidents that led you to understand your status as a patient in a new way and conclude by generalizing about your insight.

Draw a character sketch: after using physical as well as psychological details, end by explaining how this person has enhanced or damaged the quality of your life.

Sustain a dialogue: present your topic through two distinctively different voices engaging with each other and coming to agreement or disagreement.

Begin with a quotation: unpack the significance of an especially evocative passage or a wrongheaded expert opinion that can be better understood through some aspect of your condition.

Start with a generalization or an aphorism: analyze how an incident in the progress of your disease or treatment either substantiates or undercuts it.

Explain how to do something: set out the specific steps it takes to complete a process that you have had to undertake or found beneficial (for example, physical therapy for lymphedema or a prosthetic limb).

Elaborate on an abstract term: consider your cancer experience in terms of a concept like mercy or clarity.

Contrast before and after: describe how a medical intervention or conversation changed you physically or psychologically.

Extend an analogy: defy Susan Sontag's prohibition against metaphors by comparing an illness experience with an entirely different realm of experience and then consider how the analogy holds up or breaks down.

Annotate a list: should you, for instance, tackle platitudes, present what people say to cancer patients in a list annotated with your editorial comments.

Collect a mini-archive: analyze a cancer-related phenomenon in the media (such as pharmaceutical ads, TV hospital commercials, or the absence of attention to a disease like bladder cancer).

Appropriate an alternative lexicon: use a vocabulary from a field unrelated to cancer (sports or religion, say) to explore some aspect of your experience of disease.

Add your two cents: discuss a typical cancer problem (the scar, hair loss) as it is presented in the reading you have done and then explain how your experience compares with the experiences of others.

Question a frequently used term (like "survivor" or "terminal") or a cliché ("cancer makes us cherish the present moment") and revitalize it or make it obsolete.

Coin a new word (like "scanxiety" or "chemoflage") and explain why it is needed.

Begin with an email you received that sparked your response and then elaborate on what you did or did not write back.

Push the envelope by articulating what you feel has not yet been articulated by other patients or by medical authorities.

Push the envelope because only you can explain what you have encountered, endured, and understood.

Did I mention pushing the envelope?

Actually, I have no idea what "pushing the envelope" literally means or where this phrase comes from—I don't fancy asking Siri—but it seems exactly right. I don't know how you will do it, but I do know that it has to be and will be done. I really do know that, if nothing else.

For me, one avenue that provided an escape from the tug-of-war between self-censorship and self-expression came naturally. Unlike many people who blog about illness, I have been trained as a scholar of the arts and therefore wanted to disclose not only my own experiences of cancer but also my encounters with visual art and imaginative writing. More, I wanted to use literature and art to illuminate the struggles of cancer patients. In other words, I wanted to sneak in the humanities.

As a teacher and a reader, I have used the poetry of Gerard Manley Hopkins to understand the misery of insomnia, the verse of Emily Dickinson to clarify the anguish of intense pain, and a villanelle by Elizabeth Bishop to elucidate the various losses that any serious diagnosis presages. Quoting verse in a scholarly book entails time-consuming and frustrating paperwork to determine ownership, not to mention payments to obtain permission. But the editors at the *Times* never bothered with such matters, and even whole stanzas of poems were reproduced without burdensome paperwork or expenses.

If artists without cancer can create work that helps people understand the disease and its treatment, what might artists with cancer produce? That question sent me on numerous treasure hunts. When I found the paintings of Robert Pope, who died from Hodgkin's disease in 1992, and Hollis Sigler, who died from breast cancer in 2001, I worried that TPP would not want to devote space to artwork. She hired me, after all, to discuss my life with cancer. But like many cancer patients, I spend an inordinate amount of time alone—alone, that is, with books and the Web. If I could articulate how these paintings enriched my understanding of my life with cancer and also addressed the fears and hopes of other patients, I would be helping to create an archive of cancer art.

I was delighted to take advantage of the appearance of a film version of the wonderful young adult novel *The Fault in Our Stars* to write a piece about the book. Since children generally cannot record their own cancer experiences, fiction plays a unique role in suggesting what they may be undergoing. And without suppressing the suffering that cancer entails, John Green's novel illuminates the precocity that miserable treatments can paradoxically grant adolescents. This essay, about a novel composed about (not by) a person dealing with terminal cancer, helped me broaden the parameters of the cancer canon. In all these cases, I felt that the blog functioned a bit like notes for a lecture.

As the role of blog writer melded with that of English teacher, I inevitably turned to memoirs, graphic novels, and creative nonfiction. However, my engagement could not be that of a traditional literary critic. A formal analysis or cultural studies approach was not to my purpose: I needed to show what literature could tell me and my readers about our disease. Indeed, when I submitted a piece on the biblical book of Job, it was rejected, and I knew the fault was my own. Exploring the complexity of this exceptionally ironic text had not left me enough space to integrate it into a personal framework.

With other works, I did find various ways to highlight an issue in my life. For example, Miriam Engelberg's graphic memoir *Cancer Made Me a Shallower Person* analyzes a divide in the breast cancer population between those with a primary diagnosis and those with metastatic disease; I contrasted that division with my experience of advanced ovarian cancer as a chronic condition that may be neither curable nor terminal. Similarly, the grief of a child in Judith Vaninstenael's graphic novel *When David Lost His Voice* could punctuate a description of my attempts to help my adult daughters deal with my future demise.

When I look over the accumulated blogs of "Living with Cancer," it seems to me that they fall into four categories: (1) personal experiences, (2) patient quandaries, (3) epistemological haze, and (4) the healing arts. Three of these are self-evident, but by "epistemological haze" I mean all the columns in which I kept on coming up against forms of unknowingness: of our bodies, of the causes of cancer, of when there is a recurrence, of other people about the nature of our disease, of how to estimate our odds or make impossibly difficult medical and economic and familial decisions, of where the cancer is spreading, of dying and death. The most rewarding columns enabled me to protest medical wrongs: misdiagnosis, especially of young adults, and negligent care, especially of people suffering from incurable disease. From the start, the blogs gave me an opportunity to address my fears of dying and my sorrow at death.

The act of mourning propelled a succession of elegies I composed on the cancer deaths of friends. Each was undertaken because of a keen sense of loss; however, I tied each to a societal issue pertinent to a large population of patients. In this regard, they illustrate my efforts to meld the four categories, integrating personal experience not only with the arts but also with patient quandaries and epistemological haze.

So, for instance, I discussed environmental causes of cancer in the elegy for my graduate student; the importance of palliative care and hospice in the elegy for a member of my support group; and in the elegy for a cherished colleague, the challenge of moving beyond anger to a sense of peace while dying. Only later did I understand this sort of project as part of what the anthropologist S. Lochlann Jain has called "elegiac politics." Jain rejects a politics of disavowal (survivorship), a politics of cheerfulness (the pink ribbon), and a politics of denying suffering (drives for a cure). Like Jain, I feel that translating private grief into the public realm places death and dying at the center of the cancer experience—which is, sadly, exactly where they do reside.

The extensive reading as well as the privilege of being able to honor those living and dying with cancer buoyed me up throughout the beginning of 2013, the year that my oncologist predicted would be my last. As exhilarating as it was to be writing about living with cancer, some antediluvian part of me still believed that what "counts" as a publication is a printed book. In May 2013, therefore, I sent an email to the senior editor John Stickney, asking about the possibility of my reprinting the blogs, or a selection of them, in a book.

He responded, "The standard agreement—the one you signed last year—means that you and the NYT share half the proceeds from any book comprised exclusively of your columns." Whether or not that fact would inhibit my agent from trying to peddle such a project, John Stickney's email somehow liberated me from my book fixation. After all, a simple Web search of my name produces all the essays as well as the readers' responses. Isn't that as much of an afterlife as the one achieved by the tomes I have published, many of which have been remaindered?

How strange that a relinquished wish can be fulfilled in an unforeseen manner! For then I drafted a column called "Writing Therapy," which generated a proposal titled *Writing Cancer*—and the result is the book you have in your hands (from which the *Times* has generously relinquished all rights). I am greatly indebted to the column for prompting me to search far and wide for an archive that constitutes an evolving cancer tradition that I have tried to chart in these pages.

Paradoxically, though, the blog has convinced me of the virtues of the printed book. For only in this decidedly less interactive and longer format can I quote other scholars who have enriched my thinking, qualify or extend my arguments, dare to reveal more honestly my qualms, broach the problem of speaking truthfully about the body, explore the formal as well as the cultural dimensions of literature, and reiterate the occasional curse word.

Undoubtedly, though, the column has instructed me on the potential of the Internet for patient advocacy. On the Web, cancer blogs and message boards proliferate: patients ask and answer all conceivable questions, describe their treatments, and explore ways of alleviating the consequences of the disease and its medical protocols. YouTube contains innumerable lectures by medical specialists, testimonials by patients, demonstrations by nurses, and interviews of caregivers that assist many people with often stigmatized problems. The speed and reach of information help patients and caregivers find not only answers but a sense of community. When Charles Harris confronted metastasized colon cancer, he found blogging "a godsend": "The blog became talking therapy," in part because responses from his family and friends made him feel "less isolated than I have ever been in my life."

Looking back on my various struggles with the column, though, I realize that I have been resisting the blog's implicit promise to report up-to-the-minute particulars of its author's quotidian existence. Why should the specificities of my life be more significant than those of anyone else's? The issue goes beyond my efforts to protect my and my circle's privacy, for I am constantly attempting to make the blog more capacious, less self-referential. It is the egotism of the genre that troubles me.

Given the interactive format of the blog, this might seem like a strange claim. For it is certainly the case that after individual readers regularly posted month after month, I began to appreciate their predicaments. Some found my email address and communicated directly with me in letters or sent me manuscripts-in-progress, to which I responded because they moved me with their valiant insights into disease. Since my university affiliation is available on the Web, others mailed me an astonishing assortment of gifts: handmade greeting cards, books of poems and of photographs, T-shirts emblazoned with logos of nonprofit organizations they had founded, book bags, hand creams, pins, CDs, and DVDs.

Needless to say, I tried to thank all these individuals. But it seemed wrong to comment on posted replies in the blog itself. Although, before cancer forced me to retire, I relished back-and-forth conversations and debates with students even in a large lecture hall, on the website I felt as if I had had my say and the comments section belonged to the readers. In part, too, I would not call the sort of blog I composed truly interactive, because I had no idea whether, how, or on what basis the *Times* blocked or filtered unacceptable comments from readers.

Maybe it is the illusion of interactivity that underscored for me the imbalance between the author—absorbed in the particularities of her circumstances—and readers, who react with little or no expectation of being answered. On other sites, ingenious authors managed to be much more personally responsive than I. A blogger named Leroy Sievers, for example, engaged in discussions with readers on the NPR webpage "My Cancer." From 2006 until a few days before his death in 2009, he not only encouraged readers to react to his posts about treatment for metastatic colon cancer but quoted them and wrote back to them on the site.

Still, bloggers are supposed to place themselves front and center, and sometimes they do so for questionable purposes, namely selling a load of products while branding themselves. Consider the self-promotion of Kris Carr's blog on my.crazysexylife.com— "home of the crazysexywellnessrevolution"—which can be browsed by categories: "how to nourish and heal your body," "restore your mind and spirit," "empower your lifestyle," and "align your words and passion." Marketing her girl-power identity, Kris Carr also produced a series of books to give cancer a makeover and in the process take in what Lorrie Moore would call a big wad o' cash.

To my mind, the controversy swirling around one noncommercial and quite serious blog by Lisa Bonchek Adams crystalizes more complex problems related to blogging and self-disclosure. At age 37, Lisa Adams was diagnosed with and treated for breast cancer. She continued writing about her family and her treatments after she suffered a recurrence. Her posts about metastatic disease were especially disturbing, as she declined while a series of aggressive protocols were tried and failed and others were started. At the start of 2014, two journalists—Emma Gilbey Keller and Bill Keller—published related, though quite different, critiques of the blogs. In a January 8 post on the *Guardian*'s U.S. website, Emma Keller wondered whether electronic disclosures on chronic disease or terminal care constitute TMI (too much information). In particular, she called Lisa Adams's tweets "a grim equivalent of deathbed selfies." Bill Keller, partly to defend his wife's column, used Lisa Adams (in a January 12 *New York Times* op-ed) to criticize Americans who deploy every possible technology to wage war against cancer and stave off death, unlike the British, who accept palliative care.

Most readers agreed that Bill Keller had missed the mark. Lisa Adams sought not to exploit but to question military hype about bravely battling against and then winning victory over breast cancer. She pursued treatments for metastatic disease, fully aware that they would not cure her, and she did so, in part, because she wanted to live as long as possible with and for her three young children. She died in March 2015. Also, since I believe that Americans have increasingly come to understand the benefits of palliative care, Bill Keller's criticism strikes me as unfounded. His wife's essay led to such appalled responses that the *Guardian* removed it from the Web. Yet Emma Keller had raised a thorny issue. The idea of producing cancer selfies—surgery selfies, radiation selfies, chemo selfies, hospice selfies—revolts me too.

There is no doubt that the instantaneous speed and the geographical breadth of personal revelations circulating on the Internet can breed exhibitionism in writers, while provoking voyeurism in readers. I think Lisa Adams avoided the pitfalls of delivering the electronic equivalent of a macabre reality TV show, as I hope I have, but such hazards nevertheless threaten to contaminate good—by which

I mean stimulating, educative, thoughtful—communications. In today's tell-all culture, the digital blogger tends—under the pressure of frequent postings—to record more and reflect less than the diarists of the past. Reflection about an event often requires the passage of a considerable amount of time, which frees a person to transform its meaning retrospectively. In a book on the history of diaries, Alexandra Johnson claims that "bloggers have assumed the mantle of traditional diary keeping—the daily entry—reinventing it in the process." She also enumerates numerous software options for diarists in the digital age, such as Diary Book, Diary Defender, Alive Diary, Advance Diary, Personal Diary, Efficient Diary, My Voice Diary, and Anxiety Diary.

But the equation of the blog with the diary entry disregards not only the quick pace of posting but also the public nature of cyberspace for essays that can be emailed, tweeted, and uploaded onto Facebook; it also discounts the influence of readers' comments, which have absolutely no analogue in the traditionally kept diary of old. Because of these factors, I never viewed my blogs as diary entries. By my lights, the most jejune feelings and events are diary-worthy; however, I wanted to post blogs only about issues that concern many other cancer patients. When widely disseminated, every word on emotionally charged topics such as inflated drug costs, failed trials, and insurance glitches has the capacity to trigger painful memories, defensive rebuttals, or angry reactions in readers. I therefore had to work through umpteen revisions of each essay. All the spontaneity of the diary evaporated.

While writing this chapter, I realized that many forms of my self-censorship are related to this anxiety not about self-promotion but about a self-centeredness that inadvertently misrepresents or marginalizes other people's experiences and thereby inflicts dam-

age. I wanted to write in a way that would lead beyond my own out-
look on my cancer and would speak to people with quite different
vantages on theirs. It has been easier to ward off exhibitionism than
the tendency to generalize from my personal experience in a way
that fails to take into account how partial and limited my singular
perspective must be.

One way around all these minefields involved my taking on
the role of a compassionate witness. As memoirs and stories about
cancer suggest, compassionate witnessing can help unlock feelings
in people made rigid by fear and pain. When I wrote about the
suffering of friends, the composition process certainly released my
own feelings of grief. At times, oddly, literary criticism and theory
became a means of compassionate witnessing, as I sympathized
with various characters or voices in the works of poets and fiction
writers or quoted the astute words of such thinkers as Nancy K.
Miller and Eve Kosofky Sedgwick. (I wonder if a blog hinged on
my identification with the characters in Bernardine Bishop's novel
*Unexpected Lessons of Love* would liberate me from generalizing
about my distressed reaction to the ostomy.)

I also tried to stretch the genre of the blog by discussing books
about the scientific, medical, and economic problems retarding
research or compounding the quandaries of patients. I guess you
can take the teacher out of the classroom, but you can't take the
classroom out of the teacher.

Perusing cancer sites daily, I sometimes worry that the *Times* task
means that my remaining months or years will be consumed by
the disease. Instead of reading and writing about cancer, shouldn't

I be taking advantage of this reprieve by traveling, bonding with my grandchildren, moving with my husband into a smaller house or apartment, making a bucket list (as in a kick-the-bucket list) of what I want to accomplish before my death? Truth be told, writing has always been a (if not the) supreme pleasure in my life. And this sort of writing helps me keep track of what I am feeling and learning. Now that I have lost sight of Suleika—she has stopped posting in order to follow other pursuits—I harbor a fantasy of reaching out to her through email, to thank her for being such an inspiring muse.

Back in 2008, at diagnosis, my oncologist worried that a promising drug in the pipeline might not be available (even in trial form) soon enough to extend my life. I also had read that Phase I clinical trials, using drugs never before tested on human beings, try to establish the right dosage and do not generally benefit patients; in fact, these drugs can harm or even kill them. I could never have predicted that I would be kept alive by a Phase I clinical trial or by writing for the *Times*. And so, dragging and kicking my feet, I've been converted little by little to precisely the optimistic sort of approach to cancer that used to infuriate me. Given my anxiety about cancer selfies, I do not know what I will do when the experimental pills fail to keep my cancer at bay. Will "Living with Cancer" morph into "Dying with Cancer"? Or by that time, will I have run out of steam? Will the benefits of composing and posting have come to an end?

Or perhaps readers will lose interest, if I don't start dying sooner rather than later! This suspicion plagued a wonderful columnist for the London *Times*, John Diamond, who in the late 1990s reported on the progress of his throat cancer. With astonishing clarity, he described the operations that removed chunks of his tongue and the resulting shock of voicelessness. Viewing himself as a "honking dribbler," he worried that he "was no longer the person my friends befriended, my wife married." The husband of the food writer Nigella Lawson, Diamond explained how he felt receiving all nourishment through a feeding tube, and he mourned the father-loss their two young children would inevitably suffer. He wanted to face reality without becoming a drag and worried that reports of his demise might be greatly exaggerated: "What if I carry on for years, having told everyone that the end is nigh? How embarrassing would that be?" I knew I had found a kindred spirit when he wrote, "Everyone who gets the cancer diagnosis should be given a national newspaper column by way of therapy." Like him, I was lucky to receive that gift.

I still understand that advanced ovarian disease is incurable and I continue to decry barbaric treatments. But the clinical trial in which I am enrolled—with a targeted drug far superior to poisonous chemotherapy—not only extends my life but also gives me time that I can savor. Four pills taken daily at home make it possible for me to attribute the unforeseen gift of my ongoing existence not to cancer but to pioneering medical research. The surprising extension of my life has deepened my awareness of mutability and mortality and of the need to appreciate and testify to life as it is lived. To say thank you also for the blog, I have decided to close this book with a revision of one of my posts, because its sentiments continue to reflect my conviction that reading and writing have an amazing capacity to buoy hale spirits in frail bodies.

When with a wild surmise I watched my November 2013 birthday approach, arrive, and recede, I said to a friend then dying from cancer, "It feels weird to be living on borrowed time." She responded, "You'll have to come up with a better term for it."

Yes, "borrowed time" does sound parsimonious as a label for the unearned bounty of more time and a decidedly thicker earthly existence than I had ever expected. It also sounds silly: borrowed from whom and to be paid back how? I have read of patients surviving beyond what they call their "expiration date," but that implies that the life left was spoiled or rancid.

The better term surfaced in a poem by Raymond Carver about a man told eleven years earlier that he had six months to live unless he quit drinking and who then somehow sobered up:

> After that it was all gravy, every minute
> of it, up to and including when he was told about,
> well, some things that were breaking down and
> building up inside his head. "Don't weep for me,"
> he said to his friends. "I'm a lucky man.
> I've had ten years longer than I or anyone
> expected. Pure Gravy. And don't forget it."

Working and loving and being loved, Raymond Carver's seasoned speaker finds new ways to be sauced in his second life—even after the onset of terminal disease.

The sociologist Arthur W. Frank, admiring the same poem, believes that "Gravy is beyond health or illness, beyond the desire for health, which necessarily brings the fear of the illness. Gravy does not romanticize illness but is willing to accept it for what it can bring." Like Raymond Carver's dying speaker, I harbor no illusions about a cure: I know that a longer period of remission is all I can hope for. The death sentence has not been commuted but stayed— deferred not by any efforts on my part but by the sheer luck of access to an unpredictably effective drug. Nor do I want my exultation at beating the odds to erase or disrespect those people, many of them cherished friends, whose deaths established the grim statistics.

Yet this November 2014 and throughout the next month and then the next in 2015, I have continued to relish the anticipation of another posting, fervent outrage about a work retitled or a paragraph slashed, keen gratitude for a thrilling illustration, future struggles to tell difficult truths about the body, and acute curiosity about the tender as well as tendentious responses of readers who have become a challenging audience and, in my wildest dreams, a virtual community. For my lack of control over some aspects of "Living with Cancer" reflects my lack of control over living with cancer, which, in turn, teaches me about, yes, our abiding and inevitable lack of control.

I finish this book with gratitude that I was given sufficient time to do so and with hope that the time granted its readers will be filled with more reading and writing. Counting from now back to the predicted prognosis death date, I picture myself as a lurching one-and-a-half-year-old, savoring pure gravy, every minute of it. Even if I don't reach two or three or four, I have had my delicious share.

# Notes and Suggested Readings

PREFACE. NOTES

2 Virginia Woolf, *On Being Ill*, introduction by Hermione Lee (Ashfield, Mass.: Paris Press, 2002), p. 21.

7 Woolf, *On Being Ill*, pp. 3–4.

8 Samantha King coined the phrase "The Tyranny of Cheerfulness" in the subtitle of chapter 5 of *Pink Ribbons, Inc.: Breast Cancer and the Politics of Philanthropy*.


CHAPTER 1. NOTES AND SUGGESTED READINGS

11 The quotation from E. M. Forster is actually from one of his characters. In *Aspects of the Novel* (New York: Harcourt Brace Jovanovich, 1985), he quotes this question asked by "the old lady in the anecdote who was accused by her nieces of being illogical" and who was "really more up to date" than her educated relatives (p. 101).

14 Esther Dreifuss-Kattan, *Cancer Stories: Creativity and Self-Repair* (Hillsdale, N.J.: Analytic Press, 1990), p. 3.

15 Elizabeth Bishop's "One Art" can be read online in its entirety.

17 W. H. Auden was quoted in a 1970 magazine article (*Life*, January 30, 1970, p. 54); the aphorism is by the Austrian writer Karl Kraus.

17 Judith Guest, foreword to *Writing Down the Bones: Freeing the Writer Within*, by Natalie Goldberg (Boston: Shambhala, 1986), p. xii.

17 Joan Didion, "Why I Write," in *Essays and Conversations*, ed. Ellen G. Friedman (Princeton: Ontario Review Press, 1984), p. 6.

18 Arthur W. Frank, *At the Will of the Body: Reflections on Illness* (Boston: Houghton Mifflin, 1991), p. 2.

18 Anatole Broyard, *Intoxicated by My Illness* (New York: Clarkson Potter, 1992), pp. 23–24.

18 Matt Freedman, *Relatively Indolent but Relentless: A Cancer Treatment Journal* (New York: Seven Stories Press, 2014), n.p. This book reproduces the pictorial journal, unpaginated, that Freedman kept in the fall of 2012.

18 Dan Shapiro, *Mom's Marijuana: Life, Love, and Beating the Odds* (New York: Vintage Books, 2000), p. 84.

18 John Diamond, *C: Because Cowards Get Cancer Too . . .* (London: Vermilion, 1998), p. 10.

18 Le Anne Schreiber, *Midstream* (New York: Viking, 1990), pp. 10–11.

19 The work of James W. Pennebaker, published in *Opening Up: The Healing Power of Expressing Emotions* (London: Guilford Press, 1997 [a revised edition of *Opening Up: The Healing Power of Confiding in Others* (1990)]), is described by Louise DeSalvo in *Writing as a Way of Healing: How Telling Our Stories Transforms Our Lives* (Boston: Beacon Press, 2000), p. 19.

19 Pennebaker, *Opening Up*, pp. 34, 40.

19 DeSalvo, *Writing as a Way of Healing*, p. 9.

20 Jeffrey Wolin collects his portraits of survivors in *Written in Memory: Portraits of the Holocaust*. For more on trauma studies in relation to the Holocaust, see Shoshana Felman and Dori Laub's *Testimony: Crises of Witnessing in Literature, Psychoanalysis, and History*.

20 Siddhartha Mukherjee, *The Emperor of All Maladies: A Biography of Cancer* (New York: Scribner, 2010), p. 398.

20 Dreifuss-Kattan, *Cancer Stories*, pp. 130, 125, 129.

21 Kathrin Milbury et al., "Randomized Controlled Trial of Expressive Writing for Patients With Renal Cell Carcinoma," *Journal of Clinical Oncology* 32 (2014): 663, 667.

22 Anne Hunsaker Hawkins, "Writing about Illness: Therapy? Or Testimony?," in *Unfitting Stories: Narrative Approaches to Disease, Disability, and Trauma*, ed. Valerie Raoul, Connie Canam, Angela Henderson, and Carla Paterson (Waterloo, Ont.: Wilfrid Laurier University Press,

2007), p. 123. In this essay, Hawkins cautions against the obsessive narcissism of writing that can perpetuate trauma. In addition to programs like Visible Ink and Hawkins's program at Penn State, the journal *Lifelines*, produced by the Geisel School of Medicine at Dartmouth, offers a space for writers to share literature and poetry that combines art and medicine. More information can be found at http://geiselmed.dartmouth.edu/lifelines/about/.

22 Tara Parker-Pope discusses research on revising life stories and improving self-perceptions; in "Writing Your Way to Happiness" (*New York Times*, January 10, 2015), she recommends Timothy D. Wilson's *Redirect: Changing the Stories We Live By*.

23 Rudyard Kipling, "Surgeons and the Soul" (1923), in *A Book of Words* (New York: Charles Scribner's Sons, 1928), p. 237. Kipling was considering how words can narcotize people, but they can also stimulate them.

23 Graham Greene, *Ways of Escape* (New York: Simon and Schuster, 1980), p. 10.

23 On free writing, see the work of Peter Elbow, *Writing without Teachers* (New York: Oxford University Press, 1973), as well as Pat Schneider, *Writing Alone and with Others* (New York: Oxford University Press, 2003), and Lynn Lauber, *Listen to Me* (New York: W. W. Norton, 2004). The quotations in this paragraph are from Lauber, p. 61, and Schneider, p. xx.

24 Elbow, *Writing without Teachers*, p. 136.

24 Sharon Bray provides weekly writing prompts for people dealing with disease at www.writingthroughcancer.com

26 Elbow, *Writing without Teachers*, p. 18.

28 Gwendolyn, in act 2 of Oscar Wilde's *The Importance of Being Earnest*, in *The Norton Anthology of English Literature: The Victorian Age*, general editors M. H. Abrams and Stephen Greenblatt, ed. Carol T. Christ, 7th ed. (New York: W. W. Norton, 2000), vol. 2B, p. 1790.

28 "Death is the mother of beauty" is from "Sunday Morning," in *The Collected Poems of Wallace Stevens* (New York: Knopf, 1954), p. 68.

28 Virginia Woolf, *A Writer's Diary* (Orlando, Fla.: Mariner Books, 2003), p. 13.

30 Doris Lessing is quoted in Herbert Mitgang, "Mrs. Lessing Addresses Some of Life's Puzzles," *New York Times*, April 22, 1984.

31   Kathlyn Conway, *Ordinary Life: A Memoir of Illness* (New York: W. H. Freeman, 1997), p. 2.

31   René Magritte's *La trahison des images* (1929, *The Treachery of Images*) is in the collection of the Los Angeles County Museum of Art, Los Angeles, and can be viewed at LACMA.org. "Not Ideas about the Thing but the Thing Itself," in *The Collected Poems of Wallace Stevens*, p. 534.

32   Edward Said, *Reflections on Exile and Other Essays* (Cambridge, Mass.: Harvard University Press, 2000), p. 566. In the preface to his memoir *Out of Place* (New York: Knopf, 2000), Said tells the reader, "Several years ago I received what seemed to be a fatal medical diagnosis, and it therefore struck me as important to leave behind a subjective account of the life I lived in the Arab world, where I was born and spent my formative years, and in the United States, where I went to school, college, and university" (p. xi). At the start of *Bathsheba's Breast*, a history of breast cancer, James S. Olson explains that his treatment for a soft-tissue sarcoma led to his writing the book.

32   Oliver Sacks, "My Own Life," *New York Times*, February 19, 2015.

33   Musa Mayer, *Examining Myself: One Woman's Story of Breast Cancer Treatment and Recovery* (Boston: Faber and Faber, 1993), p. 6.

34   On writing as a way for patients to gain control, see Thomas G. Couser, *Recovering Bodies: Illness, Disability, and Life-Writing*.

34   On Rachel Carson, see Sharon Batt, *Patient No More: The Politics of Breast Cancer*. Nora Ephron's son, Jacob Bernstein, explained his mother's reasons for choosing to keep her leukemia a secret in "Nora Ephron's Final Act," in the *New York Times Magazine*, March 10, 2013. After Carolyn Heilbrun's death, Susan Kress provided a new conclusion to her biography, *Feminist in a Tenured Position*.

34   Henry James, *The Wings of the Dove* (New York: Modern Library, 2003), pp. 267, 257, 441, 374.

35   Anne Lamott, *Bird by Bird: Some Instructions on Writing and Life* (New York: Pantheon Books, 1994), p. 19.

36   For a history of journal writing, see Alexandra Johnson, *A Brief History of Diaries: From Pepys to Blogs* (London: Hesperus Press, 2011). Johnson explains the number of best-selling diaries by women: "Centuries of prohibition and inhibition had driven women to diary keeping. Safe yet secret" (p. 59).

36 Fanny Burney, *The Diary and Letters of Madame D'Arblay*, in *The Norton Anthology of Literature by Women: The Traditions in English*, ed. Sandra M. Gilbert and Susan Gubar, 3rd ed. (New York: W. W. Norton, 2007), 1:350–57; I quote from this edition because it is the most accessible. According to Dina Rabinowitch, "Not until the 1890s were surgeons willingly using anaesthesia on every patient": *Take Off Your Party Dress: When Life's Too Busy for Breast Cancer* (London: Pocket Books, 2007), p. 48. Of course the scene of mastectomy is missing in most contemporary memoirs, but Juliet Wittman observes another woman's mastectomy at the end of her memoir *Breast Cancer Journal: A Century of Petals*.

37 "He, also, sought then": Burney, *The Diary and Letters*, p. 351.

37 "Too sympathizing partner": Burney, *The Diary and Letters*, p. 353.

37 When Burney finally receives: Burney, *The Diary and Letters*, p. 354.

38 Burney's lengthy letter: Burney, *The Diary and Letters*, pp. 354, 351, 353.

38 But her (and my): Burney, *The Diary and Letters*, p. 351.

38 All the coming-and-going characters: Burney, *The Diary and Letters*, pp. 353–56.

39 *The Diary of Alice James*, ed. Leon Edel (New York: Dodd, Mead, 1964), pp. 206–7. Also see Ruth Bernard Yeazell's excellent introduction to *The Death and Letters of Alice James: Selected Correspondence*, ed. Yeazell. A contemporary author who felt "something like relief, even elation" at diagnosis is Anatole Broyard, who experienced the first stage of illness as "a rush of consciousness, a splash of perspective, a hot flash of ontological alertness": *Intoxicated by My Illness*, pp. 3, 7.

40 Resentful that her doctors dismissed her ills: *Diary of Alice James*, p. 211.

41 Surely Alice James knew: *Diary of Alice James*, pp. 208, 225.

41 One of Alice James's: *Diary of Alice James*, p. 226.

41 Valuing not the extension of her life: *Diary of Alice James*, pp. 229, 230.

42 Alice James dictated to her companion: *Diary of Alice James*, p. 232.

42 Paradoxical to the end: *Diary of Alice James*, p. 232.

43 Broyard, *Intoxicated by My Illness*, p. 61.

43 Audre Lorde, *The Cancer Journals* (San Francisco: Spinsters/Aunt Lute, 1980). See also Lorde's account of dealing with metastatic disease in *A Burst of Light*.

44 In the first reprinted journal entry: Lorde, *The Cancer Journals*, p. 11.

44 In her retrospective, essayistic prose: *The Cancer Journals*, pp. 31, 38.

44 Throughout *The Cancer Journals*: Lorde, *The Cancer Journals*, pp. 36, 42.

45 Audre Lorde bristles: Lorde, *The Cancer Journals*, pp. 60, 59, 60.

46 Already out of the closet: Lorde, *The Cancer Journals*, pp. 16, 70.

46 Even in the italicized journal entries: Lorde, *The Cancer Journals*, pp. 76, 77.

47 *Hollis Sigler's Breast Cancer Journal*, with texts by Susan M. Love, M.D., and James Yood. For a scholarly appreciation, see Laura E. Tanner, "Living Breast Cancer: The Art of Hollis Sigler," *Tulsa Studies in Women's Literature* 32.9/33.1 (Fall 2013/Spring 2014): 219–39.

47 Benedict B. Benigno, *The Ultimate Guide to Ovarian Cancer* (Atlanta: Sherryben Publishing House, 2013), p. 217.

48 William Strunk Jr. and E. B. White, *The Elements of Style*, 4th ed. (New York: Longman, New York, 1999), p. xviii; Stephen King, *On Writing: A Memoir of the Craft* (New York: Scribner, 2000).

49 The Purdue Online Writing Lab, http://owl.english.purdue.edu/owl/.

Decades ago, I faced freshmen bored by handbooks. I therefore created a handout to remind them about the most frequent grammar errors made by writers of all ages and stages.

### HERES HOW TO REALLY KNOW IF YOU WRITE GOOD

1. Make each pronoun agree with their antecedent.
2. About those sentence fragments.
3. When dangling, watch your phrases.
4. Verbs has to agree with their subjects.
5. Don't be to proud to use a dictionary.
6. Avoid run-on sentences, they are hard two read.
7. Just among you and I, case is important.
8. Try to not ever split infinitives.
9. Proofread your work to see if any words out.
10. Use the virtuous word for your meaning.
11. Students misuse of the possessive apostrophe is as widespread as there misuse of "its."
12. For the most part a common follows an introductory element.

The joke here, of course, is that each entry contains at least one and sometimes more than one mistake. (Students were asked to circle twenty mistakes on the handout.)

49 James Thomas, "How to Write a Sentence," *New Yorker* online, October 24, 2014.

49 King, *On Writing*, p. 123.

49 Christopher Hitchens, "Unspoken Truths," *Vanity Fair*, June 2011, p. 50; he attributes the writing advice to the *Guardian* writer Simon Hoggart.

50 King, *On Writing*, p. 117.

51 Alberto Barrera Tyszka, *The Sickness*, trans. Margaret Jull Costa (London: Quercus, 2010), p. 130.

52 S. Lochlann Jain created the word "chemoflage," in *Malignant: How Cancer Becomes Us* (Berkeley: University of California Press, 2013), p. 183.

52 Eve Kosofsky Sedgwick, "Advanced Degree: School Yourself in Resilience to Beat Depression," Off My Chest column, *Mamm Magazine*, September 2000, p. 24.

53 On Facebook, Britany Maynard posted a final goodbye to readers on November 1, 2014.

54 Randy Pausch wrote *The Last Lecture* (New York: Hyperion, 2008) with Jeffrey Zaslow. The video of the lecture, titled "Really Achieving Your Childhood Dreams," has been archived online by Carnegie Mellon at www.cmu.edu/randyslecture/.

54 Christopher Hitchens, *Mortality* (New York: Twelve, 2012), pp. 43, 44.

55 Jane Catherine Lotter, "Jane Catherine Lotter Obituary," *Seattle Times*, July 28, 2013; available online at www.legacy.com/obituaries/seattletimes/.

55 Kafka is quoted in Nicholas Murray, *Kafka* (London: Little, Brown, 2004), p. 343.

56 Truman Capote, *Truman Capote: Conversations*, ed. N. Thomas Inge (Jackson: University Press of Mississippi, 1987), p. 38.

56 E. L. Doctorow, quoted in Bruce Weber, "The Myth Maker," *New York Times Magazine*, October 20, 1985. Doctorow also noted, "I've discovered that you cannot start a book with an intention, a calculation. You start writing before you know what you want to write or what it is you're doing."

56  Joyce Carol Oates, "Selections from a Journal: January 1985–January 1988," in *Private Lives: Journals, Notebooks, and Diaries*, ed. Daniel Halpern (Hopewell, N.J.: Ecco Press, 1998), p. 332.

56  Annie Dillard, *The Writing Life* (New York: Harper Perennial, 2013), pp. 11, 68.

The many books about using a journal and free writing for personal growth include Kathleen Adams, *Journal to the Self*; Christina Baldwin, *One to One*; Sharon A. Bray, *When Words Heal*; Natalie Goldberg, *Old Friend from Far Away* and *The True Secret of Writing*; Linda Trichter Metcalf and Tobin Simon, *Writing the Mind Alive*; and James W. Pennebaker, *Writing to Heal*. The cancer survivor Barbara Abercrombie has produced two books for patients: *Writing Out the Storm: Reading and Writing Your Way through Serious Illness or Injury* and *Courage & Craft: Writing Your Life into Story*.

Janet Burroway explains how to turn journal entries into short stories in *Writing Fiction: A Guide to Narrative Craft*. For books on how to write stories and narratives more generally, including creative fiction and nonfiction, see William Zinsser, *How to Write Well*; Richard Rhodes, *How to Write: Advice and Reflections*; Victoria Mixon, *The Art and Craft of Fiction*; Priscilla Long, *The Writer's Portable Mentor: A Guide to Art, Craft, and the Writing Life*; Jonathan Franklin, *Writing for Story: Craft Secrets of Dramatic Nonfiction*; and Mark Kramer and Wendy Call, eds., *Telling True Stories: A Nonfiction Writers' Guide from the Nieman Foundation at Harvard University*.

If you're interested in illustrating your stories, Scott McCloud's *Making Comics* has excellent tips. For books focusing on how to write poetry rather than narrative fiction, see Mary Oliver, *A Poetry Handbook*; Ted Kooser, *The Poetry Home Repair Manual: Practical Advice for Beginning Poets*; John Drury, *Creating Poetry*; John C. Goodman, *Poetry: Tools & Techniques, a Practical Guide to Writing Engaging Poetry*; and Kim Addonizio, *Ordinary Genius: A Guide for the Poet Within*. For interviews with famous authors on their experiences of writing, their writing process, and how they write, see the *Paris Review* series "The Art of Poetry," "The Art of Fiction," and "The Art of Comics."

## CHAPTER 2. NOTES AND SUGGESTED READINGS

58 Anthony Hopkins, playing C. S. Lewis, speaks this line in William Nicholson's script for *Shadowlands*, directed by Richard Attenborough (HBO Home Video, 1999), DVD.

58 Marcel Proust, *On Reading*, ed. Jean Autret and William Buford (New York: Macmillan, 1971), p. 55.

59 Will Schwalbe, *The End of Your Life Book Club* (New York: Vintage, 2013), p. 7.

59 Quotations from Job are taken from *The HarperCollins Study Bible*, ed. Wayne A. Meeks et al. (New York: HarperCollins, 1993).

60 Susan Sontag, *Illness as Metaphor and AIDS and Its Metaphors* (New York: Picador, 2001), pp. 57, 3.

60 Stephen Jay Gould, "The Median Isn't the Message," in *The Richness of Life: The Essential Stephen Jay Gould*, ed. Stephen Rose (New York: W. W. Norton, 2007), pp. 27, 29, 30. This essay has been widely reproduced and can be easily accessed online.

61 Sontag, *Illness as Metaphor*, pp. 3–4. On both Susan Sontag and Stephen Jay Gould, see the excellent scholarly work of Ann Jurecic, *Illness as Narrative*. I am distinguishing the memoir focused on illness from the more wide-ranging autobiography that recounts an entire life and may also deal with cancer. See, for example, Lucy Grealy's *Autobiography of a Face*, which deals with repercussions of an operation on her jaw when she was nine years old.

63 Michael Korda, *Man to Man: Surviving Prostate Cancer* (New York: Random House, 1996). On prostate cancer, see also Robert O. Beatty with his family, *Still a Lot of Living: Coping with Cancer*. In *Wrestling with the Angel: A Memoir of My Triumph over Illness* (New York: W. W. Norton, 1990), Max Lerner confronts two cancers—lymphoma and prostate cancer. An exception to the mainly white-authored memoirs that predominate in this tradition, the Reverend Charles R. Williams and Vernon A. Williams's *That Black Men Might Live: My Fight against Prostate Cancer* (Roscoe, Ill.: Hilton Publishing, 2003) is composed for the African American community "because we black American men have a higher incidence of prostate cancer and are more likely to die from this disease" (p. xvi).

63 Vivien Gornick, *The Situation and the Story: The Art of Personal Narrative*.

63 *Discovery and detection*: Korda, *Man to Man*, p. 31.

64  *Finding and initiating treatment*: Korda, *Man to Man*, pp. 120, 134.

64  *Enduring treatment*: Korda, *Man to Man*, pp. 157, 177.

65  *Distress over bodily dysfunction*: Korda, *Man to Man*, pp. 183–84, 251.

66  In his reactions: Korda, *Man to Man*, pp. 151, 171, 189.

66  Because at the end of his memoir: Korda, *Man to Man*, pp. 57, 187, 240.

67  Throughout *Man to Man*: Korda, *Man to Man*, pp. 176, 212, 93.

68  Arthur W. Frank, *The Wounded Storyteller: Body, Illness, and Ethics* (Chicago: University of Chicago Press, 1995), p. 115. Frank contrasts the quest story both to the restitution narrative so prominent in popular culture, which showcases a triumphant return to health, and to the chaos narrative, which details the breakdown of language during intense suffering. Another useful book on illness narratives is Anne Hunsaker Hawkins, *Reconstructing Illness: Studies in Pathography*.

68  Through one landmark book at the start of this tradition, a memoirist changed medical practices. Rose Kushner's writings sparked widespread criticism of the radical Halsted operation as well as a "one-step" approach to breast cancer that was then standard practice: a tumor biopsy and mastectomy performed in a single operation while the patient was under anesthesia. Kushner, wanting patients to exert some control over treatment decisions, was booed off the stage at the Society of Surgical Oncology in 1975, the year she published her memoir, *Why Me? What Every Woman Should Know about Breast Cancer to Save Her Life*. But in 1990 she was posthumously awarded the Society's James Ewing Award for outstanding contributions to the fight against cancer. On the historic role played not only by Rose Kushner's memoir but also by Betty Rollins's *First, You Cry*, see Barron H. Lerner, M.D., *The Breast Cancer Wars: Fear, Hope, and the Pursuit of a Cure in Twentieth-Century America*, and James S. Olson, *Bathsheba's Breast*.

68  Anatole Broyard, *Intoxicated by My Illness* (New York: Clarkson Potter, 1992), pp. 47, 54, 57.

69  Barbara Creaturo, *Courage: The Testimony of a Cancer Patient* (New York: Pantheon, 1991), pp. 147, 145, 156, 250.

70  Marianne A. Paget, *A Complex Sorrow: Reflections on Cancer and an Abbreviated Life* (Philadelphia: Temple University Press, 1993), p. 20. Her earlier sociological study of medical errors is titled *The Unity of Mistakes*.

70  S. Lochlann Jain, *Malignant: How Cancer Becomes Us* (Berkeley: University of California Press, 2013), pp. 49–50, 107.

70  Reynolds Price, *A Whole New Life* (New York: Scribner Classics, 2000), pp. 50, 56, 93, 96, 144–45, 145, 99.

71  That traditionally trained specialists remain: Price, *A Whole New Life*, pp. 109, 141, 183. In *The New Cancer Survivors: Living with Grace, Fighting with Spirit*, Natalie Davis Spingarn also criticizes conventional doctors for only giving her more pain pills, and she attempts to use hypnosis, the Feldenkrais method, biofeedback machines, and acupuncture to deal with treatment-related pain.

72  Le Anne Schreiber, *Midstream* (New York: Viking, 1990), pp. 138, 120.

72  Schreiber, *Midstream*, pp. 163–64; Gerda Lerner, *A Death of One's Own*.

73  Simone de Beauvoir, *A Very Easy Death*, trans. Patrick O'Brian (New York: Pantheon Books, 1985), p. 82.

73  Stan Mack, *Janet & Me: An Illustrated Story of Love and Loss* (New York: Simon and Schuster, 2004), pp. 10, 81, 145, 146. Stewart Alsop describes a period in the early 1970s when physicians at NIH prescribed martinis for him and derided the fact that many other physicians told a person with acute leukemia "only that he has anemia" so "he is not hopelessly unhappy"; *Stay of Execution: A Sort of Memoir* (Philadelphia: J. B. Lippincott, 1973), pp. 71–72. Perhaps the most disturbing memoir about denial is David Rieff's *Swimming in a Sea of Death*, for with distressing ambivalence the son of Susan Sontag must collude with her denial of a blood cancer that killed her after her two earlier aggressive battles against breast and uterine cancer.

73  Allen Widome, *The Doctor/The Patient: The Personal Journey of a Physician with Cancer* (Miami: Editech Press, 1989), p. 147.

74  Edward E. Rosenbaum, *A Taste of My Own Medicine: When the Doctor Is the Patient* (New York: Random House, 1988), pp. 52, 189, 214, viii. Other physician-patient memoirs include Geoffrey Kurland, M.D., *My Own Medicine*, and Samuel Sanes, M.D., *A Physician Faces Cancer in Himself*.

74  Fitzhugh Mullan, M.D., *Vital Signs: A Young Doctor's Struggle with Cancer* (New York: Farrar Straus Giroux, 1983), pp. 20, 47, 129, 486.

75  Mullan, *Vital Signs*, p. 160.

75 Janet R. Gilsdorf, M.D., *Inside/Outside: A Physician's Journey with Breast Cancer* (Ann Arbor: University of Michigan Press, 2006), pp. 174, 217.

75 Katherine Russell Rich, *The Red Devil: To Hell with Cancer—and Back* (New York: Crown Publishers, 1999), pp. 38, 168.

75 Amanda Bennett, *The Cost of Hope* (New York: Random House, 2012), pp. 177, 223.

76 Evan Handler, *Time on Fire: My Comedy of Terrors* (New York: Little, Brown, 1996), pp. 46, 196, 194–95, 235. Martha Fay has produced a markedly different perspective in a study of eight patients at Memorial Sloan-Kettering in *A Mortal Condition*. Robin Roberts praises the staff at Memorial Sloan-Kettering for providing precisely the compassionate witnessing she needed when she felt herself "slipping away" during a bone marrow transplant for myelodysplastic syndrome, caused by earlier chemotherapy for breast cancer; Roberts with Veronica Chambers, *Everybody's Got Something* (New York: Grand Central Publishing, 2011), p. 164.

77 Handler, *Time on Fire*, p. 177.

77 Dan Shapiro, *Mom's Marijuana: Life, Love, and Beating the Odds* (New York: Vintage, 2000), p. 89.

77 Eve Ensler, *In the Body of the World: A Memoir* (New York: Henry Holt, 2013), pp. 71, 83.

77 The memoirist quoted is Kathlyn Conway, *Ordinary Life: A Memoir of Illness* (New York: W. H. Freeman, 1997), p. 107.

78 Evan Handler, *It's Only Temporary: The Good News and the Bad News of Being Alive* (New York: Riverhead Books, 2008), pp. 96, 97.

78 Adam Wishart, *One in Three: A Son's Journey into the History and Science of Cancer* (New York: Grove Press, 2007), p. 149.

78 Emily Dickinson, "My Life had stood - a Loaded Gun," F. 764 / J. 754.

79 The first-century Talmudic scholar Hillel (*Pirkei Avot* 1:14).

80 Gordon Stuart is quoted in Arthur Kleinman, *The Illness Narratives: Suffering, Healing, and the Human Condition* (New York: Basic Books, 1988), p. 148.

80 Alicia Ostriker, "Scenes from a Mastectomy," in *Living on the Margins: Women Writers on Breast Cancer*, ed. Hilda Raz (New York: Persea, 1999), p. 181.

80 Siddhartha Mukherjee, *The Emperor of All Maladies: A Biography of Cancer* (New York: Scribner, 2010), p. 38.

80 Lynn Kohlman, *Lynn Front to Back* (New York: Assouline Publishing, 2005). This coffee-table book is not paginated. The striking warrior photograph, shot by Mark Obenhaus, appears right after Donna Karan's foreword; it is juxtaposed to a photograph of a youthful Kohlman with breasts.

81 Christina Middlebrook, *Seeing the Crab: A Memoir of Dying before I Do* (New York: Doubleday, 1996), pp. 75, 2, 77, 85, 81.

81 Although scared, the boy-soldier: Middlebrook, *Seeing the Crab*, pp. 56, 61, 72, 62.

82 John Diamond, *C: Because Cowards Get Cancer Too . . .* (London: Vermilion, 1998), pp. 192–93, 72.

82 See Suzanne Somers, *Knockout: Interview with Doctors Who Are Curing Cancer—and How to Prevent Getting It in the First Place*; Patrick Quillin, *Beating Cancer with Nutrition*; Anne E. Frahm and David J. Frahm, *A Cancer Battle Plan*; William L. Fischer, *How to Fight Cancer and Win*; Tamara St. John, *Defeat Cancer Now: A Nutritional Approach to Wellness for Cancer and Other Diseases*; and Richard C. Frank and Gale V. Parsons, *Fighting Cancer with Knowledge and Hope: A Guide for Patients, Families, and Health Care Providers*.

83 Deborah Cumming, *Recovering from Mortality: Essays from a Cancer Limbo Time* (Charlotte, N.C.: Novello Festival Press, 2005), pp. 13, 54.

83 Arthur W. Frank, *At the Will of the Body: Reflections on Illness* (Boston: Houghton Mifflin, 1991), p. 83.

84 See "And Beth Shall Be No More—*Little Women*, Heroines, and Nora Ephron," the July 30, 2014, blog on *Oblomov's Sofa*: http://oblomovssofa.wordpress.com/

84 Cumming, *Recovering from Mortality*, p. 46.

84 Kathy Acker, "The Gift of Disease," *The Guardian–Weekend*, January 1997, pp. 14, 16.

84 Ruth Picardie, *Before I Say Goodbye: Recollections and Observations from One Woman's Final Year* (New York: Henry Holt, 1998), p. 97; Dina Rabinovitch, "We've Had War, We've Had Plagues, but Never This . . . ," *Guardian*, October 21, 2007.

85  Ensler, *In the Body of the World*, p. 38; Joyce Wadler, *Cured, My Ovarian Cancer Story* (Greensboro, N.C.: e-Quality Press, 2013), p. 25.

85  George Johnson, *The Cancer Chronicles: Unlocking Medicine's Deepest Mystery* (New York: Vintage Books, 2014), pp. 35, 82, 91, 68.

86  See *Exploding into Life* (New York: Aperture, in association with Many Voices Press, 1986), pp. 44, 50, a collaboration between Dorothea Lynch and the photographer Eugene Richards that documents her breast cancer treatments and cancer care in Boston-area hospitals.

86  Juliet Wittman, *Breast Cancer Journal: A Century of Petals* (Golden, Colo.: Fulcrum Publishing, 1993), pp. 4, 174.

87  Lerner, *Wrestling with the Angel*, pp. 63, 50, 51.

87  Barbara Ehrenreich, *Bright-Sided: How the Relentless Promotion of Positive Thinking Is Undermining America* (New York: Henry Holt, 2009), p. 20.

87  Catherine Lord, *The Summer of Her Baldness: A Cancer Improvisation* (Austin: University of Texas Press, 2004), p. 18.

88  Lord, *The Summer of Her Baldness*, p. 189.

88  See Betty Rollins, *First, You Cry*; Lance Armstrong, *It's Not about the Bike*; Jill Ireland, *Life Wish*; Barbara Barrie, *Don't Die of Embarrassment: Life after Colostomy and Other Adventures*; Fran Drescher, *Cancer Schmancer*; and Robin Roberts, *Everybody's Got Something*.

88  Gilda Radner, *It's Always Something* (New York: Simon and Schuster, 1989), pp. 12, 140, 123, 130, 135, 228. Musa Mayer also finds herself "living in a state of perpetual envy and longing . . . for my own lost self, as I used to be," in *Examining Myself: One Woman's Story of Breast Cancer Treatment and Recovery* (Boston: Faber and Faber, 1993), p. 121.

89  Robert Schimmel with Allan Eisenstock, *Cancer on Five Dollars a Day\* (\*Chemo Not Included): How Humor Got Me through the Toughest Journey of My Life* (Cambridge, Mass.: Da Capo Press, 2008), pp. 14, 68, 71, 80, 92, 99.

89  Soon after Tig Notaro was diagnosed with breast cancer, she opened her stand-up comedy set at a Los Angeles club called Largo by announcing, "Hello, I have cancer. How are you?" She then delivered what the comedian Louis C.K. has described as "one of the greatest standup performances I ever saw" ("About Tig Notaro," October 5, 2012, *Louis CK*, http://buy.louisck.net/news/about-tig-notaro). Jenny Allen's one-woman show, *I Got Sick Then I Got Better*, satirizes

friends' responses to her cancer (for the trailer, see her website, www
.jennyallenwrites.com/promoters/). See also *Dead and Breathing*, a
play by Chisa Hutchinson.

90 Joni Rodgers, *Bald in the Land of Big Hair: A True Story* (New York:
HarperCollins, 2001), pp. 24, 45, 56.

90 The wisecracking stops: Rodgers, *Bald in the Land of Big Hair*, pp. 149,
133.

91 There really is a *Chicken Soup for the Breast Cancer Survivor's Soul*.

91 Instead of a chronological account: Rodgers, *Bald in the Land of Big
Hair*, pp. 30, 75, 77.

91 Tania Katan, *My One-night Stand with Cancer* (New York: Alyson
Books, 2005), pp. 1, 63, 88–89, 92.

92 Tania waits in a medical waiting area: Katan, *My One-night Stand with
Cancer*, pp. 108, 109, 111, 137, 178–79.

92 At the happily-ever-after ending: Katan, *My One-night Stand with
Cancer*, pp. 259, 262.

92 Katan, *My One-night Stand with Cancer*, p 262; Dina Rabinovitch,
*Take Off Your Party Dress: When Life's Too Busy for Breast Cancer* (London: Pocket Books, 2007), p. 42. For more on BRCA and on elec-
tive mastectomy, see the suggested readings at the end of this chapter's
notes.

93 For scholarly responses to cancer comics, see the suggested readings at
the end of this chapter's notes.

93 Miriam Engelberg, *Cancer Made Me a Shallower Person: A Memoir in
Comics* (New York: Harper, 2006). On issues related to "pink-washing,"
see Ehrenreich, *Bright-Sided*; Gayle A. Sulik, *Pink Ribbon Blues: How
Breast Cancer Culture Undermines Women's Health*; and Samantha King,
*Pink Ribbons, Inc.: Breast Cancer and the Politics of Philanthropy*.

94 Brian Fies, *Mom's Cancer* (New York: Abrams Comicarts, 2006), p.
18. The most famous memoir about the effects of cancer on a family is
John Gunther's best-selling *Death Be Not Proud*, about his son's struggle with and death from a brain tumor.

95 Later, in the midst of treatment: Fies, *Mom's Cancer*, pp. 59, 66.

95 Marisa Acocella Marchetto, *Cancer Vixen: A True Story* (New York:
Knopf, 2006), pp. 34–35.

96 On another page, Marchetto has drawn: Marchetto, *Cancer Vixen*, pp.
36–37.

97 Subsequent drawings embellish: Marchetto, *Cancer Vixen*, pp. 150, 156, 164, 196–97.

97 S. L. Wisenberg, *The Adventures of Cancer Bitch* (Iowa City: University of Iowa Press, 2009), pp. 45, 61.

98 David Small, *Stitches: A Memoir* (New York: W. W. Norton, 2009). In a prose memoir about her Haitian background, *Brother, I'm Dying*, Edwidge Danticat describes an uncle who survived throat cancer with an artificial voice box.

98 Midway through *Stitches*: Small, *Stitches*, pp. 182, 191, 204, 135.

99 Only a kindly psychiatrist: Small, *Stitches*, pp. 277, 287, 286.

99 Drawings of the teenager David: Small, *Stitches*, pp. 302, 324.

100 Rachel Carson's *Silent Spring* has been reprinted with an introduction by Al Gore (New York: Houghton Mifflin, 2002); Terry Tempest Williams, *Refuge: An Unnatural History of Family and Place* (New York: Vintage Books, 1991), pp. 195, 214, 283. In *A Wild, Rank Place: One Year on Cape Cod*, David Gessner is inspired by Thoreau to write about his responses to nature in the context of his testicular cancer and his father's death from lung cancer.

100 Williams, *Refuge*, p. 183.

101 Sandra Steingraber, *Living Downstream: An Ecologist Looks at Cancer and the Environment*. In a documentary with the same title, Steingraber chronicles her personal struggles as a survivor of bladder cancer. Also see the breast cancer memoirs *Manmade Breast Cancers*, by Zillah Eisenstein, and *The Wounded Breast*, by Evelyn Accad. In *Teratologies*, Jacky Stacey embeds her personal account within a cultural study of cancer.

101 Christian Wiman, *My Bright Abyss: Meditation of a Modern Believer* (New York: Farrar, Straus and Giroux, 2013), pp. 14, 30, 148. The final chapter in Christian Wiman's *Ambition and Survival: Becoming a Poet* also explores the relation of poetry to spiritual belief. Another academic who subordinates the illness narrative to a larger quest for spiritual knowledge is the philosopher Gillian Rose; see *Love's Work: A Reckoning with Life*.

102 A poet, Wiman takes issue: Wiman, *My Bright Abyss*, pp. 55, 56, 119, 128. "Sunday Morning," in *The Collected Poems of Wallace Stevens* (New York: Knopf, 1954), p. 68.

102 Not belief, but faith: Wiman, *My Bright Abyss*, pp. 139, 146, 149, 155.

103 Eve Kosofsky Sedgwick, *A Dialogue on Love* (Boston: Beacon Press, 1999), pp. 5, 15, 69.

103 Sedgwick, *A Dialogue on Love*, pp. 168, 216–17, 207. Sandy Boucher writes about confronting colon cancer with traditional medicine and Buddhist meditation in her memoir *Hidden Spring*.

104 Eve Kosofsky Sedgwick, "Pedagogy of Buddhism," in her *Touching Feeling: Affect, Pedagogy, Performativity* (Durham: Duke University Press, 2003), pp. 173, 179, 174; she discusses "the art of loosing" in "Living with Advanced Breast Cancer," *Mamm*, May 2001, not paginated.

104 Sedgwick, *A Dialogue on Love*, p. 7.

In *For All That Has Been: Time to Live and Time to Die*, Jane Cameron explores how her social work with hospice patients prepared her to deal with metastatic disease. In *A Way to Die*, Victor and Rosemary Zorza write about their daughter's dying from melanoma in hospice. Marie de Hennezel's *Intimate Death* recounts her experiences with the terminally ill in Paris. The best book on decision making during end-of-life care for cancer patients is Atul Gawande's *Being Mortal*.

For a scholarly analysis of the significance of BRCA to the definition of Jewish identity, see Jessica Mozersky, *Risky Genes: Genetics, Breast Cancer and Jewish Identity*. A helpful book for women dealing with genetic risk is *Confronting Hereditary Breast and Ovarian Cancer: Identify Your Risk, Understand Your Options, Change Your Destiny*, by Sue Friedman, Rebecca Sutphen, and Kathy Steligo.

On inherited cancers and the decision to opt for prophylactic mastectomy, see the memoirs of Janet Reibstein, *Staying Alive: A Family Memoir;* Elizabeth Bryan, *Seeing the Life: A Family in the Shadow of Cancer*; and Jessica Queller, *Pretty Is What Changes*, as well as the essay on them by Mary K. DeShazer in her *Mammographies: The Cultural Discourses of Breast Cancer Narratives*. Angelina Jolie has published a number of essays in the *New York Times* about her prophylactic surgeries.

On the comics of Brian Fies, Miriam Engelberg, and Marisa Acocella Marchetto, see Martha Stoddard Holmes, "Cancer Comics: Narrating Cancer through Sequential Art," *Tulsa Studies in Women's Literature* 32.2/33.1 (Fall 2013/Spring 2014): 147–62, as well as Nancy K. Miller, "The Trauma of Diagnosis: Picturing Cancer in Graphic Memoirs," *Configurations* 22.2 (Spring 2013): 207–23.

For other graphic memoirs, see Tom Batiuk, *Lisa's Story: The Other Shoe*; Matt Freedman, *Relatively Indolent but Relentless: A Cancer Treatment Journal*; Joyce Brabner and Harvey Pekar, illustrations by Frank Stack, *Our Cancer Year*; Alesia Shute, with illustrations by Nathan Lueth, *Everything's Okay: A Round Table Comic*; and Stan Mack, *Janet & Me: An Illustrated Story of Love and Loss*.

Another mutation in the cancer memoir involves the emergence of collaborative memoirs. See, for instance, Barbara Rosenblum and Sandra Butler's *Cancer in Two Voices* as well as Victoria Zacheis Greve and Karen Greve Young's *Love You So Much: A Shared Memoir*.

## CHAPTER 3. NOTES AND SUGGESTED READINGS

106 David Jay's photographs can be viewed online at thescarproject.org or in his book *The SCAR Project (Breast Cancer is Not a Pink Ribbon, Volume 1)*. Patricia Zagarella has produced a documentary film that follows Jay's work on this project, *Baring It All* (PBS, 2011).

107 On the subject of "unled lives" or the lives we might have lived, I am indebted to the thinking of Andrew H. Miller, who writes extensively about counterfactual histories in fiction, poetry, and film.

107 On the sublime, see Edmund Burke, *A Philosophical Enquiry into the Origin of Our Ideas of the Sublime and Beautiful*, as well as *The Sublime: From Antiquity to the Present*, edited by Timothy M. Costelloe, which includes clarifying essays not just on Burke but also on Immanuel Kant and such postmodern thinkers as Jean-François Lyotard, Gilles Deleuze, and Fredric Jameson.

107 Harold Bloom, *The Daemon Knows: Literary Greatness and the American Sublime* (New York: Spiegel and Grau, 2015), p. 6.

108 Anatole Broyard, *Intoxicated by My Illness* (New York: Clarkson Potter, 1992), p. 12.

109 Leo Tolstoy, "The Death of Ivan Ilych," in *Tolstoy's Short Fiction*, ed. and trans. Michael R. Katz, Norton Critical Edition, 2nd ed. (New York: W. W. Norton, 2008), pp. 83–128; Tillie Olsen, "Tell Me a Riddle," in *The Norton Anthology of Literature by Women: The Traditions in English*, ed. Sandra M. Gilbert and Susan Gubar, 3rd ed. (New York: W. W. Norton, 2007), 2:660–86.

111 Besides feeling guilty: Tolstoy, "Ivan Ilych," pp. 104, 110.

111 Although Ivan initially is locked: Tolstoy, "Ivan Ilych," p. 109.

111 Sheer terror: Tolstoy, "Ivan Ilych," pp. 111, 113, 114.

112 In my early teaching days: Tolstoy, "Ivan Ilych," p. 127.

112 How very curious: Tolstoy, "Ivan Ilych," p. 128.

113 No longer capitalized as "*It*": Tolstoy, "Ivan Ilych," pp. 109, 128.

113 Joanne Trautmann Banks, "Death Labors," *Literature and Medicine* 9 (1990): 162–71; E. M. Forster, "What I Believe," in *Two Cheers for Democracy* ([London]: Edward Arnold, 1951), p. 73. For "death's delirium," see Jesse Matz, "The Art of Time, Theory to Practice," *Narrative* 19 (2011): 282.

114 A fascinating analogy: Tolstoy, "Ivan Ilych," pp. 127, 110.

114 During his suffering and despite his graying beard: Tolstoy, "Ivan Ilych," pp. 115, 121, 122, 124.

115 The temporal and spatial confusion: Tolstoy, "Ivan Ilych," pp. 127, 128.

115 Elizabeth Kübler-Ross discusses the five stages of grief in *On Death and Dying: What the Dying Have to Teach Doctors, Nurses, Clergy and Their Own Families.*

115 The sublime has often been seen as a "moribund aesthetic," rather than an aesthetic of the moribund; see Thomas Weiskel, *The Romantic Sublime: Studies in the Structure and Psychology of Transcendence* (Baltimore: Johns Hopkins University Press, 1976), p. 6.

116 Before her cancer is diagnosed: Olsen, "Riddle," pp. 663, 667.

116 After an operation: Olsen, "Riddle," pp. 668, 669.

116 Because sickness incapacitates Eva: Olsen, "Riddle," pp. 670, 674.

117 At a turning point: Olsen, "Riddle," pp. 677, 676.

117 Unable to reconcile: Olsen, "Riddle," p. 678.

117 When Eva takes to her deathbed: Olsen, "Riddle," pp. 680, 682, 683.

118 Eva's singing of the socialist hymn: Olsen, "Riddle," p. 683.

118 The last paragraph: Olsen, "Riddle," pp. 686, 676.

119 "*Death deepens the wonder*": Olsen, "Riddle," p. 686.

120 Epicurus, *Letter to Menoeceus* 275, translated in James Warren, *Facing Death: Epicurus and His Critics* (Oxford: Clarendon Press, 2004), p. 19: "when we are, death is not present; and for the time when death is present, we are not." A contemporary novel about cancer by Abby Frucht, *Life Before Death*, experiments with the sort of deathbed time traveling that engrossed Tolstoy and Olsen.

121 Hannah Wilke, *Intra Venus* (New York: R. Feldman Fine Arts, 1995);

a number of the images in this series can be viewed online. On the art of Hannah Wilke, see Einat Avrahami, *The Invading Body: Reading Illness Autobiographies*, and Catherine Lord, *The Summer of Her Baldness: A Cancer Improvisation* (Austin: University of Texas Press, 2004), p. 92.

122 Esther Dreifuss-Kattan discusses Ferdinand Hodler in *Cancer Stories: Creativity and Self-Repair.*

122 Robert Pope, *Illness & Healing: Images of Cancer*, 10th anniversary ed. (Hantsport, N.S.: Robert Pope Foundation, 2002). Many of his works can be viewed on the Web.

123 In *Radiation*, for example: Pope, *Illness & Healing*, p. 53.

124 In paintings with other figures: Pope, *Illness & Healing*, pp. 58, 70.

125 "Like a dagger": Pope, *Illness & Healing*, p. 99.

126 Margaret Edson, *Wit*, in Gilbert and Gubar, eds., *Norton Anthology of Literature by Women*, 2:1454–87; quotation, p. 1472. For an example of the ovarian cancer patient as a stereotypical barren old maid, see W. H. Auden, "Miss Gee," in his *Selected Poems*. On *Wit* and other texts about dying in the hospital, see "Technologies of Dying," chapter 8 of Sandra M. Gilbert's *Death's Door: Modern Dying and the Ways We Grieve*.

127 Only during her dying: Edson, *Wit*, p. 1485.

127 "If you think eight months": Edson, *Wit*, p. 1476.

128 J. M. Coetzee, *Age of Iron* (New York: Penguin, 1990), p. 145.

128 Seeing the police: Coetzee, *Age of Iron*, pp. 64, 65, 82.

129 For most of Mrs. Curren's letter: Coetzee, *Age of Iron*, p. 129.

129 Toward the end: Coetzee, *Age of Iron*, pp. 168, 198.

129 Andrew Solomon, *A Stone Boat* (London: Faber and Faber, 1994), pp. 161, 36, 98. See also his book on depression, *The Noonday Demon*, and his essay on assisted suicide, "A Death of One's Own," *New Yorker*, May 22, 1995.

130 Harry, together with his brother: Solomon, *A Stone Boat*, pp. 104–5, 140, 204.

130 "Breathtaking to watch": Solomon, *A Stone Boat*, p. 183.

131 Judith Vanistendael, *When David Lost His Voice*, trans. Nora Mahony (London: SelfMadeHero, 2012). In black and white, another graphic novel—Ben Mitchell's *Throat: Book One*—deals with a 30-year-old confronting throat cancer.

131 A conflation of ends and beginnings: Vanistendael, *When David Lost His Voice*, unnumbered opening pages, pp. 68–70.

131 Arrivals and departures: Vanistendael, *When David Lost His Voice*, pp. 172, 173.

132 In the hospital: Vanistendael, *When David Lost His Voice*, pp. 241, 242–43.

133 Amy Hempel, "In the Cemetery Where Al Jolson Is Buried" is available online.

134 Alice Munro, "Floating Bridge," in Gilbert and Gubar, eds., *Norton Anthology of Literature by Women*, 2:1026–44; quotations, p. 1039.

135 As the sun sets: Munro, "Floating Bridge," pp. 1042, 1043, 1044.

135 Musa Mayer, *After Breast Cancer: Answers to the Questions You're Afraid to Ask* (Sebastopol, Cal.: Genentech, 2003) p. 163.

136 Alice Munro, "Free Radicals," *New Yorker*, February 11, 2008, pp. 136–43; quotations, pp. 138, 139.

136 Like Nita's love of reading: Munro, "Free Radicals," pp. 140, 141, 142.

137 Anatole Broyard, *Intoxicated by My Illness* (New York: Clarkson Potter, 1992), p. 20.

137 Lorrie Moore, "People Like That Are the Only People Here: Canonical Babbling in Peed Onk," in *The Collected Stories* (London: Faber and Faber, 2008), pp. 251–83; quotation, p. 153. For other stories about cancer in this volume, see "Go Like This," "What Is Seized," "Real Estate," and "Strings Too Short to Use." On Moore's "People Like That," see also Pamela Schaff and Johanna Shapiro's "The Limits of Narrative and Cultures," *Journal of Medical Humanities* 21.1 (Spring 2006): 1–17.

The Mother's anger at the medical establishment in Lorrie Moore's story recalls the fury percolating in Peter De Vries's earlier novel *The Blood of the Lamb* (Boston: Little, Brown and Company, 1961). De Vries's father is horrified by cancer physicians who "hounded the culprit from organ to organ and joint to joint till nothing remained over which to practice their art: the art of prolonging sickness" (p. 206). The mother of another child sinks to her knees before him, "babbling incoherently": "The words came out in a stream, English, Yiddish, oaths and imprecations, blasphemies and entreaties I could not hope to reproduce. 'All they can do is kill mice!' she said in a kind of whispered scream" (p. 219). In De Vries's autobiographical novel, the suffering of innocent children triggers a crisis of faith.

138 Hospital language frightens: Moore, "People Like That," pp. 252, 254, 264.

139 When the Mother starts to pray: Moore, "People Like That," pp. 258, 259, 262, 265.

139 While the Father continually instructs: Moore, "People Like That," pp. 260, 266, 272, 274.

140 Less laughable than pathetic: Moore, "People Like That," pp. 255, 266, 276.

140 Parents' stories: Moore, "People Like That," pp. 277, 282, 283.

141 "THERE are the notes": Moore, "People Like That," p. 283.

141 Patricia Yaeger, "Consuming Trauma: Or, the Pleasures of Merely Circulating," *Journal X* 1.2 (Spring 1997): 225–51.

141 Aleksandar Hemon, "The Aquarium," *New Yorker*, June 13, 2011, pp. 50–62; quotation, p. 62.

142 "Narrative imagination": Hemon, "The Aquarium," p. 60.

142 Ezra Pound, *ABC of Reading* (New York: New Directions, 2010), p. 29.

142 William Carlos Williams, "Asphodel, That Greeny Flower," in *Asphodel, That Greeny Flower and Other Love Poems* (New York: New Directions, 1994), p. 19.

143 Maureen N. McLane, *My Poets* (New York: Farrar, Straus and Giroux, 2012), p. 126.

144 Joan Halperin, "Injunctions," in *Her Soul beneath the Bone: Women's Poetry on Breast Cancer*, ed. Leatrice H. Lifshitz (Urbana: University of Illinois Press, 1988), p. 19.

144 Alicia Suskin Ostriker, "The Mastectomy Poems," in *The Crack in Everything* (Pittsburgh: University of Pittsburgh Press, 1996), p. 85.

144 Sandra Steingraber, "Outpatient," in *Post-Diagnosis* (Ithaca, N.Y.: Firebrand Books, 1995), p. 90.

144 Pat Borthwick, "Scan," in *The Poetry Cure*, ed. Julia Carling and Cynthia Fuller (Tarset, Northumberland: Bloodaxe Books, 2005), p. 85.

144 Christian Wiman, "Witness," in *Once in the West: Poems* (New York: Farrar, Straus and Giroux, 2014), p. 72.

144 Lucia Perillo, "Needles," in *The Body Mutinies* (West Lafayette, Ind.: Purdue University Press, 1996), p. 60.

144 Susan Deborah King, "Everywoman's Lexicon of Dread, with Commentary (Minimal)," in *One-Breasted Woman* (Duluth, Minn.: Holy Cow! Press, 2007), p. 43.

144 Pat Gray, "Cancer in the Breast," in Lifshitz, ed., *Her Soul beneath the Bone*, p. 36.

144 Gustavo Pérez Firmat, "Post-Op," in *Scar Tissue* (Tempe, Ariz.: Bilingual Press, 2005), p. 3.

144 Richard M. Berlin, "Wounds," in *Secret Wounds* (Kansas City: BkMk Press at the University of Missouri–Kansas City, 2011), p. 38.

145 Lucille Clifton, "Consulting the Book of Changes: Radiation," in *The Terrible Stories* (New York: BOA Editions, 1996), p. 23.

145 Sandra M. Gilbert, "For My Aunt in Memorial Hospital," in *Emily's Bread* (New York: W. W. Norton, 1984), p. 58.

145 L. E. Sissman, "Homage to Clotho: A Hospital Suite," in *Night Music* (Boston: Houghton Mifflin, 1999), p. 129. Also see Sissman's "Dying: An Introduction," in *Dying: An Introduction*.

145 Ifor Thomas, "Poleaxed," in *Body Beautiful* (Cardigan, Wales: Parthian, 2005), p. 28.

145 Abba Kovnar, "The Windows Grow Dark," in *Sloan-Kettering: Poems*, trans. Eddie Levenston (New York: Schocken Books, 2002), p. 34.

145 Judith Hall, "Stamina," in *Anatomy, Errata* (Columbus: Ohio State University Press, 1998), p. 27.

146 C. K. Williams, "Cancer," in *Writers Writing Dying* (New York: Farrar, Straus and Giroux, 2012), p. 31.

146 Harold Pinter, "Cancer Cells," *Guardian*, March 14, 2002.

146 James Dickey, "The Cancer Match," in *The Eye-Beater, Blood, Victory, Madness, Buckhead and Mercy* (Garden City, N.Y.: Doubleday, 1970), p. 32.

146 Marilyn Hacker, "Cancer Winter," in *Winter Numbers* (New York: W. W. Norton, 1994), p. 86.

Other famous breast surgery photographs include a widely circulated image of Deena Metzer by Hella Hammid (1977), the iconic self-photograph of Matuschka, *Beauty out of Damage* (1993), and many images produced by the British photographer Jo Spence. On these as well as subsequent collections of breast cancer photographs by Art Myers, Amelia Davis, Jila Nikpays, Amy S. Blackburn, and Charlee Brodsky and Stephanie Byram, see "New Directions in Breast Cancer Photography," chapter 5 of Mary K. DeShazer's *Mammographies: The Cultural Discourses of Breast*

*Cancer Narratives.* Frank Cordelle's *The Century Project* includes visual representations of women with metastatic breast cancer. Also see the photographs of Jennifer Merendino taken by her husband, Angelo.

Many novels beyond those discussed in this chapter—starting with Peter De Vries's *The Blood of the Lamb*—integrate cancer into plots about love and death. Contemporary novels for adults include John Banville's *The Sea*, Bernardine Bishop's *Unexpected Lessons in Love*, Michael Cunningham's *The Snow Queen*, Anita Diamant's *Good Harbor*, Lucinda Ebersole's *Death in Equality*, Stanley Elkin's *George Mills*, Gail Godwin's *The Good Husband*, Nadine Gordimer's *Get a Life*, Susan Minot's *Evening*, Elizabeth Nunez's *Anna-In-Between*, Richard Powers's *Gain*, Cynthia Reeves's *Badlands*, Philip Roth's *The Dying Animal*, May Sarton's *A Reckoning*, Marshall Terry's *Angels Prostate Fall*, and Rafael Yglesias's *A Happy Marriage*.

A best seller in Europe, Ray Kluun's novel *Love Life* has been translated into English and compared to Erich Segal's *Love Story*. *The Sickness*, a novel by the Venezuelan writer Alberto Barrera Tyszka, has been translated into English, as has the French writer Pascale Kramer's *The Child*. The Swiss writer Maja Beutler has composed an autobiographical novel about the psychological impact of cancer, *Fuss Fassen*, which has not yet been translated from German.

In Iain Banks's novel *The Quarry*, the faithful caretaker of a cancer patient is an 18-year-old on the autism spectrum. Excellent young adult novels such as *The Fault in Their Stars* by John Green and *Life on the Refrigerator Door* by Alice Kuipers contextualize cancer for adolescents. Other young adult and children's novels about cancer include Jenny Dowham, *Before I Die*; Katherine Hannigan, *Ida B*; Patricia Hermes, *You Shouldn't Have to Say Goodbye*; Patrick Ness, *A Monster Calls*; Margo Rabb, *Cures for Heartbreak*; Adam Rapp, *Punkzilla*; Jordan Sonnenblick, *After Ever After*; and Holly Thompson, *The Language Inside*—and there are many more. Two young adult novels in verse—Holly Thompson's *The Language Inside* and Guadalupe Garcia McCall's *Under the Mesquite*—focus on girls dealing with their mothers' cancer. After treatment for lung cancer, Alice Trillin responded to a 12-year-old friend's cancer diagnosis by composing an advice book for children, *Dear Bruno*, illustrated by Edward Koren.

Movies about cancer include *Dark Victory*, *Bang the Drum Slowly*, *The Doctor*, *After the Wedding*, *The Shootist*, *Lightning over Water*, *Beginners*, and *Biutiful*. *American Splendor* focuses on the graphic artist

Harvey Pekar and his wife Joyce Brabner, who collaborated on a series of comic books that deal, in part, with his cancer.

To sample the evolution of the tradition of short fiction about cancer, see Margaret Atwood, "Hairball," in *Wilderness Tips*; Nina Shope, "Hangings," in *Hangings*; Nanci Kincaid, "Pretending the Bed Is a Raft," in *Pretending the Bed Is a Raft*; and Donald Antin, "The Emerald Light in the Air," in *The Emerald Light in the Air*. In *Internal Medicine*, the physician Terrence Holt tells stories that are partly fictional, partly based on his experience with patients, some of whom are cancer patients.

### CHAPTER 4. NOTES AND SUGGESTED READINGS

157  One of the most famous episodes concerning "trolls" involved Lee Siegel's blog for the *New Republic*. Negative comments led him to assume the false identity of "Sprezzatura," who championed the blog and insulted the insulters online. See Heather Armstrong's account in "The Perils of Keeping It Real," in Scott Rosenberg's collection *Say Everything: How Blogging Began, What It's Becoming, and Why It Matters*.

162  Ward Sutton, "Let's try focussing" cartoon from the *New Yorker*, February 22, 2013.

164  Virginia Woolf wrote about the unsolved problem of writing about the body in "Professions for Women," in *The Death of the Moth and Other Essays* (reprinted in *The Norton Anthology of Literature by Women*, ed. Sandra M. Gilbert and Susan Gubar).

166  Carol Chase Bjerke, *Hidden Agenda* (Madison, Wis.: Borderland Books, 2008), n.p.

167  Barbara Barrie, *Second Act: Life after Colostomy and Other Adventures* (New York: Scribner, 1997), pp. 126, 150, 226, 240.

171  Eve Ensler, *In the Body of the World* (New York: Henry Holt, 2013), pp. 52, 53.

173  Bernardine Bishop, *Unexpected Lessons in Love* (London: John Murray, 2013), p. 265. Bishop, who dealt with bowel cancer, died a few months after this book was published. For more writing on ostomies, see the suggested readings at the end of this chapter's notes.

180  S. Lochlann Jain, "Living in Prognosis: Toward an Elegiac Politics," *Representations*, no. 98 (Spring 2007): 77–92; for the passage I summarize, see p. 89. See also Jain, "Be Prepared," in *Against Health: How*

*Health Became the New Morality*, ed. Anna Kirkland and Jonathan Metzl, and Jain, "Cancer Butch," *Cultural Anthropology* 22.4 (November 2007): 501–38.

182 Charles Harris, *Incurable: A Life after Diagnosis* (Cold Spring Harbor, N.Y.: Cold Spring Harbor Laboratory Press, 2011), pp. xii, 43; this book collects his blogs. See also the website *Oblamov's Sofa* (http://oblomovssofa. wordpress.com/), where a blogger has archived her "cancer gripes" in the category "Oy vey." The MTV reality star Diem Brown blogged for People. com until 2014, when she died from ovarian cancer at age 32.

183 On Kris Carr as a postfeminist, see Emily Waples, "Emplotted Bodies: Breast Cancer, Feminism, and the Future," *Tulsa Studies in Women's Literature* 32.2/33.1 (Fall 2013/Spring 2014): 47–70.

183 See Lorrie Moore, "People Like That Are the Only People Here: Canonical Babbling in Peed Onk," in *The Collected Stories* (London: Faber and Faber, 2008), p. 264; this story is discussed above in chapter 3.

185 Alexandra Johnson, *A Brief History of Diaries: From Pepys to Blogs* (London: Hesperus Press, 2011), p. 94.

187 The first quotation from John Diamond is from *C: Because Cowards Get Cancer Too . . .* (London: Vermilion, 1998), p. 170; the others are from his London *Times* columns, which are available online.

189 Raymond Carver, "Gravy," in *All of Us: The Collected Poems*, ed. William L. Stull (London: Harvill Press, 1996), p. 292.

189 Arthur W. Frank, *At the Will of the Body: Reflections on Illness* (Boston: Houghton Mifflin, 1991), p. 140.

Gillian Rose discusses an ostomy after she reveals her diagnosis of ovarian cancer midway through her autobiographical *Love's Work*.

Only at a later time did I read a self-published ovarian cancer memoir by a woman who hated living with a colostomy and whose hernia surgeon repaired it, even though her oncologist had told her that she had to be cancer-free for two years before the colostomy could be reversed. Unfortunately, soon after the reoperation, her CA125 skyrocketed into the 1600s (a number over 35 is an indicator of cancer). See Jamie C. Schneider, *Who Will Make the Pies When I'm Gone? Living the Dark Side of Cancer (No Sugar Added)*. In a graphic memoir about a childhood diagnosis of cancer of the large intestine and colon, *Every-*

*thing's Okay* (illustrated by Nathan Lueth), Alesia Shute describes her youthful responses to an ileostomy.

On the ethics of self-disclosure in personal writing, see Thomas B. Couser, *Recovering Bodies: Illness, Disability, and Life-Writing.* On betrayal and self-betrayal, see Nancy K. Miller's *Bequest and Betrayal.* In "Memory Stains" (in *Extremities: Trauma Testimony and Community,* ed. Nancy K. Miller and Jason Tougaw [Urbana: University of Illinois Press], p. 210), she explains that "In autobiography, the acts—performed and witnessed—that might seem to beg not to be revealed are the very ones that produce writing."

# Acknowledgments

With dedication and inventiveness, my trusty research assistants—Shannon Boyer and Kelly Hanson—tracked down and discovered many texts, hauled books from and back to the library, negotiated interminably with the hassles of interlibrary loan, and facilitated my access on the Web to a plethora of material. Their queries and critiques strengthened an early draft.

Numerous colleagues and instructors have floated ideas and suggested readings that enriched my thinking on the subject of writing and cancer, especially Frank David, Ellen Dwyer, Christine Farris, Jen Fleissner, Oscar Kenshur, Lara Kriegel, Deena Lahn, Alyce Miller, Nancy K. Miller, the late Susan Moke, James Naremore, Laurie Riggins, Scott Russell Sanders, and Dr. Robert Stone. I profited enormously from the willingness of Andrew H. Miller and John Schilb to devote time to commenting on a later draft. Their careful and smart responses enriched the final manuscript.

Ongoing conversations with friends near and far have kept me in sound mind: especially Judith Brown, Shehira Davezac, Dyan Elliott, Jonathan Elmer, Mary Favret, Georgette Kagan, Jon Lawrence, Alexandra Morphet, Jan Sorby, Jayne Spencer, Mary Jo Weaver, and the late Patricia Yaeger.

Dealing with my less sound body, the brilliant oncologist Daniela Matei and her brilliant research nurse Alesha Arnold prove even to my cynical soul that exemplary health care remains a reality for some, despite our tangled system. I could never have continued working on the subject of cancer without the input and strength of Trudy Brassel, Dana Cattani, Ilka Dietrich, Carrol Krause, Julia Livingston, Traci Schmitz, and the late Leslie Wright.

The encouragement of my former collaborator, Sandra M. Gilbert, shaped this project from beginning to end. As for Tara Parker-Pope and Toby Bilanow at the *New York Times*, their unwavering responsiveness and courtesy have astonished me for many more months than I would ever have imagined.

The production of this book was facilitated by the always astute and timely interventions of my wise agent Ellen Levine; my creative editor at W. W. Norton, Jill Bialosky; and the excellent work of her assistant, Maria Rogers. It was a dream come true to have my former graduate student Alice Falk copyedit a manuscript fine-tuned not only by her scrupulosity but also by her astonishing intellect.

Most of all, I am indebted to every member of my family. The generosity of my cousins, Bernard and Colin David, never ceases to amaze me. My brother, Carl W. David, subjected himself to numerous Internet Scrabble games. Justine and Pauline, Cassie and Ben and Suneil know how much pleasure they give me.

With a heart full of love and gratitude, I say thank you for your loving-kindness and thank you again and again to my stepdaughters, Julie and Susannah Gray; to my daughters, Marah Gubar and Simone Silverbush; and to my sons-in-law, John Lyons, Kieran

Setiya, and Jeff Silverbush. As for my grandchildren—Jack, Eli, Samuel, and Jonah: you are the gravy.

When late one night I awoke my beloved husband to ask if it disturbed him that I was so engrossed with this project that for days on end I had not really taken in one word he had said, Don Gray responded, "Well, you show up at dinner." Hey, I probably retorted, who makes the dinner? But what I thought was that without his steadfast affection, companionship, humor, editorial skills, and wisdom, this book would not exist and neither would I.

# Credits